GOOD FAT IS GOOD FOR GIRLS

GOOD FAT IS GOOD FOR GIRLS

Puberty and Adolescence

DR. ELIZABETH BRIGHT

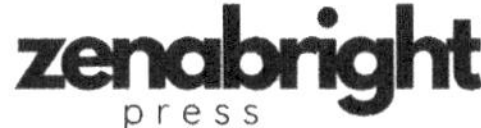

Good Fat Is Good for Girls: Puberty and Adolescence
Dr. Elizabeth Bright

ISBN: 979-8-879399-62-2

Published By Zenabright Press
www.elizbright.com

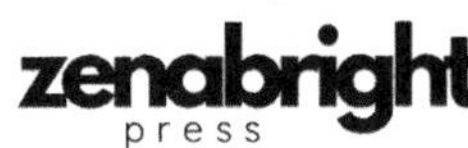

Editing by Kathy Gaudry
Book Design by Journey Bound Publishing

First Edition
Printed in the United States of America

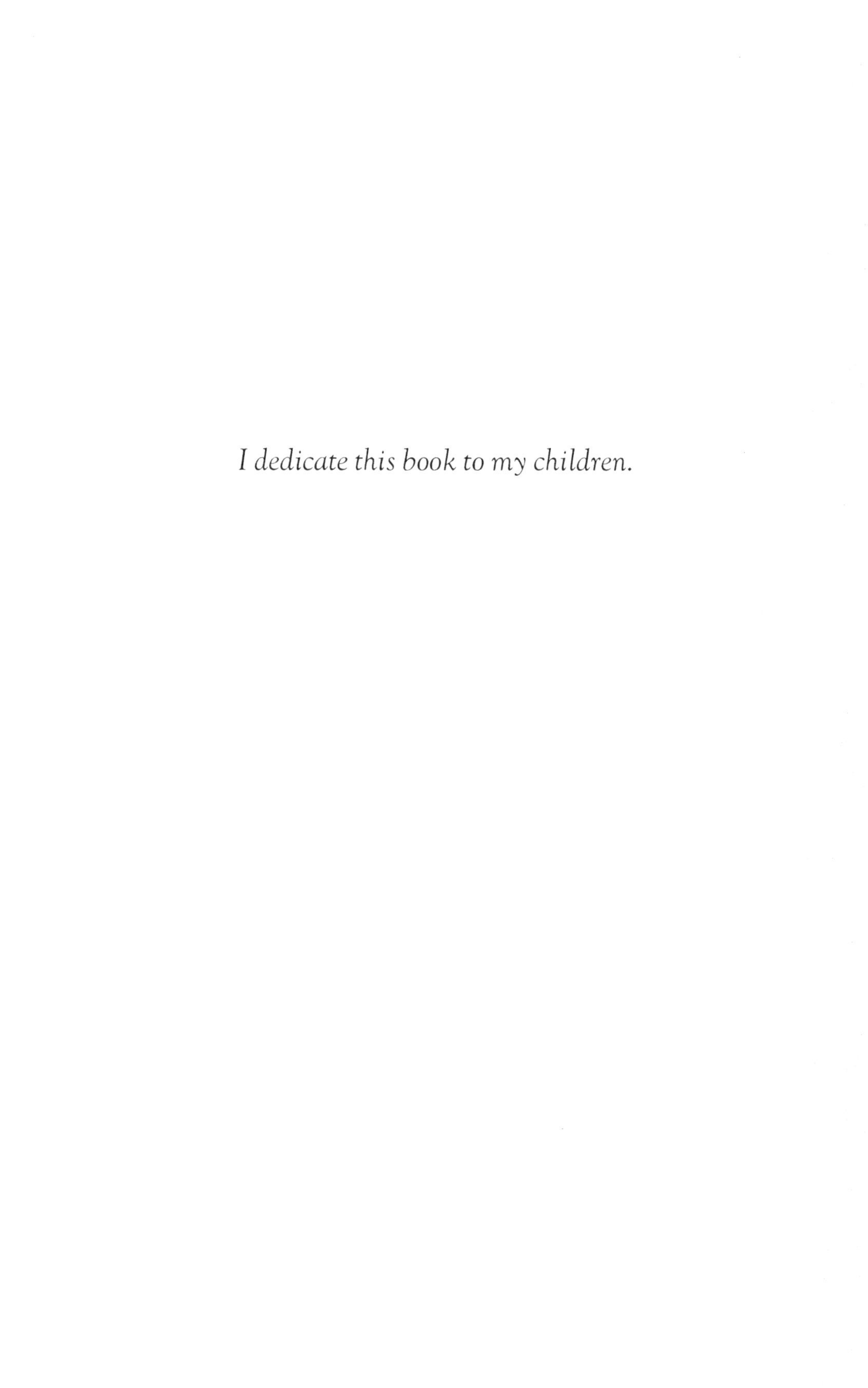

I dedicate this book to my children.

TABLE OF CONTENTS

FOREWORD

AS A BOARD-CERTIFIED HOLISTIC CARNIVORE nutritionist, finding physicians who advocate for a diet low in carbohydrates, rich in fatty meats, and supplemented with iodine is rare. My introduction to Dr. Elizabeth Bright came during an insightful discussion about thyroid health and the significance of animal fats. This discussion led me to her empowering book, *Good Fat Is Good for Women: Menopause*, which aligned with my understanding of the benefits of dietary fatty meat for optimal health. In this first book, Bright effectively debunks the common misconceptions surrounding menopause, offering a more accurate perspective on hormones and challenging the notion that menopause must be an unpleasant experience. She provides thoughtful guidance on navigating menopause healthily. Bright applies her insightful approach to adolescence and puberty in her second book, *Good Fat Is Good for Girls: Puberty and Adolescence,* offering similar clarity and understanding.

I have often used Bright's recommendations in our clinical practice to help menopausal women thrive. But how do we support young girls and boys? In her second book, Bright sheds light on the complexities and wonders of the transition from girlhood to womanhood. She articulates the journey as a unique and personal experience for each person, both influenced by various environmental and societal factors.

Bright's approach is empathetic and informative, as she includes personal vulnerabilities with scientific insights, offering a rare glimpse into the misunderstood and misinterpreted phase of female development. The book encourages a different perspective from this transition's conventional standard care purview, advocating for a more natural and holistic understanding of the changes young women undergo. This conversation is needed in a world where medication and diagnoses are often hastily and dangerously prescribed as solutions to the natural process of maturation. In fact, these "solutions" can lead to detrimental harm during a period of critical growth.

What happens when we start taking birth control pills for acne? We learn from Bright that we oftentimes use birth control pills to support hormonal imbalances stemming from nutrient deficiencies. What happens to the growing body when birth control further destroys nutrients? In my book, *Carnivore Cure*, I share how nutrients become depleted with certain pharmaceutical drugs—birth control pills lower vitamin B6, B12, folic acid, magnesium, zinc and selenium.

Pro-Tip: These nutrients are rich in meat. I wonder how many prescribing physicians mention these nutrient risks.

Bright addresses the societal and cultural influences that have shaped our perception of puberty and adolescence. She questions why society has come to view these natural changes as problematic, requiring intervention, and delves into the historical context of this perspective. This critical examination is eye-opening, revealing the commercial and societal forces contributing to a skewed understanding of young women's health. Could *creating* a problem make for a financially beneficial solution?

Bright also discusses the role of environmental factors such as xenoestrogens that impact proper development during adolescence, the importance of a nutrient-rich Carnivore diet for smooth transitions, and critical elements such as iodine in thyroid and reproductive health. The book's exploration of nutrient deficiencies, especially in modern diets and environmental factors, helps us understand how these factors impact the thyroid and overall health, leading to misdiagnosed conditions. Bright also touches on issues such as PCOS and endometriosis, highlighting how common these conditions have become and the need for a deeper understanding of their implications.

Common doesn't mean it's normal.

While it's becoming more common for menstruation to begin at an earlier age, girls starting their period at the age of eight or nine should not be considered normal. Bright argues that this early onset is often a warning sign of an imbalanced hormonal state and often comes with a higher risk of depression and anxiety. What happens when young children's cognitive, social and emotional development does not align with their age? Bright delves into the issues and offers guidance on addressing and managing them effectively.

Dr. Elizabeth Bright's book explains the physiological and hormonal changes we expect to see in females beyond definitions we can find on Dr. Google or Dr. Standard Care. *Good Fat Is Good for Girls* challenges conventional views and offers a new, holistic approach to understanding young women's health. It's a must-read for anyone seeking to understand the true nature of the transition from adolescence to womanhood and for those looking to support young women in navigating these changes with knowledge, compassion, and empowerment.

I experienced my first menstruation at the age of 13, a bit later than some of my friends. At the time, I worried that something was wrong with me, fearing that I wasn't developing properly. Soon after my period began, I noticed weight gain, which added to my confusion and prompted me to start dieting. Had I had access to this book then, I would have understood that there is no single "right" way to develop during puberty. This knowledge might have significantly reduced my insecurity and uncertainty. It could have guided me to properly nourish myself, potentially preventing the subsequent years of battling a debilitating eating disorder and frequent bouts of depression, struggles that took decades to overcome.

Judy Cho
Board Certified in Holistic Nutrition
Functional Nutritional Therapy Practitioner
Author of *Carnivore Cure* and
The Complete Carnivore Diet for Beginners

PREFACE

IF ADOLESCENCE IS NOT AN illness, why are so many medications recommended to adolescent girls during this time? Girls are prescribed twice the amount of anti-depressants than adolescent boys. Girls are prescribed hormones for various health issues unrelated to contraception. Boys are not.

Adolescents have the same health issues as younger and older women, but the difference is that at this time, sexual characteristics are being formed. Female adolescence is not an illness. In popular culture, although it is not associated with illness or decay that must be addressed with medicine as menopause is, it is still seen as a time that must be controlled and directed by medical professionals and pharmaceuticals.

I am not an adolescent. I am 61 years old. I wrote *Good Fat Is Good for Women: Menopause* because I did not want women to feel they needed to take synthetic hormones (this includes bio-identical hormones, which are also synthetic) when I knew they could address the symptoms associated with menopause by addressing adrenal function. What I learned from writing *Good Fat Is Good for Women: Menopause* gave me a particular perspective on how medicine has historically viewed women—as lesser beings whose reproductive organs are the basis of their health and well-being, both mental and physical. The same applies to female adolescents. This book is very personal for me because I have three children, two of them daughters.

The fact that a woman's clitoral anatomy was not studied adequately until the 1990s is frightening. Even more so is the fact that labiaplasty, the fastest-growing surgery worldwide, is performed by plastic surgeons who haven't even been taught the correct anatomy of the female vulva, leaving thousands of women deformed and without the ability to orgasm.

Jessica Ann Pin's work to have (at the time of this writing) 12 medical anatomy textbooks amended with proper clitoral anatomy is only one example of how science has ignored women's health because women in our culture are seen as inferior to men, dominated by biology and their reproductive organs. Researchers have described this as medical imperialism, a consequence of medical ideas that became widespread during the 19th century and led to women being easy targets for physicians and drug companies. Making a woman feel like her health issues are caused by her being female makes it easy for doctors and medical companies to make her feel she needs treatment. This book will discuss the medicalization of being a girl.

ONE

THE PERILS OF PUBERTY

WE ARE ALL WORRIED ABOUT the health of adolescent girls. Rates of depression have risen precipitously in the last ten years. Newspapers and magazines run headlines such as "Why American Teens Are So Sad"[1] in the *Atlantic*, "Teenagers are growing more anxious and depressed" in the *Economist*.[2] In *The New York Times*, "Teen Girls Report Record Levels of Sadness, C.D.C. Finds,"[3] and another, "Stop Treating Adolescent Girls as Emotionally Abnormal,"[4] because research describes this problem as being particularly associated with girls. Teenage girls are three times more likely to be depressed than boys.[5]

But it isn't only the rising rate of depression, hence mental health issues that are frequently associated with social media use, that is concerning.[6] The rate of adolescent girls suffering from polycystic ovary disease,[7, 8] endometriosis,[9, 10] and menstrual issues is also rising, making it clear that not only cultural and social changes are affecting the health of teenage girls but also physiological ones.[11] And it's the girls who suffer most. More girls than boys have both mental and physical health issues with the onset of puberty.[12]

Adolescence is defined as the period that comes between childhood and adulthood. Puberty, the formation of sexual characteristics and maturity, happens during this time. While puberty has always occurred in humans, adolescence is very new. Some literature divides puberty and adolescence this way—puberty occurs on the outside, meaning physical changes that come with sexual characteristics, such as breast development and pubic hair growth, and adolescence happens on the inside, meaning your physiology and behavior.[13, 14] This explanation is simplistic, but it demonstrates how puberty is associated with physical changes and adolescence is more associated with behavior and psychology. Puberty starts with adolescence but has a finite ending, that of fertility, where adolescence extends for several more years until a person reaches adulthood.

However, you cannot separate puberty from adolescence. All the health issues associated with puberty and adolescence are connected and driven by an imbalance in the endocrine system. Many more problems have been attached to puberty since the invention of adolescence,[15] and this continues. Adolescence used to end at 18 and 19,[16] but in the last decade, a new stage, "Emerging Adulthood," has been "discovered," a term coined by Jeffrey Jensen Arnett that extends from 18 to 25.[17] This theory comes from the scientific discovery of neuroplasticity. The brain does not finish forming until 28 years of age and regenerates throughout the entire human lifespan.[18]

Research in evolutionary development biology shows that humans are unusual in that their brain continues to develop into adulthood.[19] Adolescence and puberty are supposed to start simultaneously, but since the advent of agriculture, human females' age of puberty has plummeted. While females in hunter-gatherer societies first menstruate at 16-18, menstruation is becoming younger and younger in developed societies.[20, 21, 22] Because it has become so common, scientists aren't even calling menstruation at 8 or 9 precocious puberty anymore.[23]

This is important as physiological fitness depends on proper growth and maturation during puberty. Hormonal signaling responds to the environment.[24, 25] Nutritional deficiencies, stress, and environmental toxins will turn hormones on or off. Girls who reach puberty earlier are shorter in stature.[26] Early puberty is also associated with depression.[27] Hormones influence not only the development of sexual characteristics but also behavior. Hence, while puberty finishes with sexual maturation, the health of the adolescent is decided by their puberty.

Today, both puberty and adolescence are seen as a dangerous time for girls. Rates of depression are higher for girls than for boys.[28] Anxiety, depression, self-harm, and suicidality are rising, as are rates of prescribing drugs to treat these issues.[29, 30] Twice as many teenage girls take antidepressants than boys.[31] The comparative rates of drug treatment and medical surgeries to treat women have always been disproportionately high. This book answers why this is and how our culture got here.

Adolescence comes later in hunter-gatherer societies. The human experiment with agriculture has changed our shape, but also the rate at which we develop. For the first time in our 200,000-year history as a species, puberty comes earlier than adolescence.[32] The phenomenon that sexual maturation precedes psychosocial development only emerged 100 years ago and creates a developmental conflict.[33] Puberty involves sexual maturation, and adolescence involves learning how to become an adult.[34] In hunter-gatherer societies, which are our closest connection to our paleolithic ancestors, the age of puberty aligns more closely with the time they learn how to become adults and parents.

Childhood stress is associated with earlier puberty and the kinds of risk-taking behavior associated with adolescence.[35] Medical literature links rates of depression, anxiety, and risk-taking with puberty.[36] Risk-taking in boys is associated with behavior such as getting into fights, stealing, driving while drunk, having unprotected sex, riding a bicycle without a helmet, visiting inappropriate websites, and behavior that can endanger their physical well-being.[37] Even though the US government spends billions of dollars yearly to teach adolescents about the dangers of smoking, drug use, drinking, unprotected sex, and reckless driving, health education doesn't seem to have any impact on the rates of risk-taking.[38]

With girls, risk-taking is associated with getting sexually transmitted diseases and pregnancy. In the 1980s, developmental scientists associated this behavior with hormones. This was a continuation of George Stanley Hall's theory that adolescent behavior was driven by biology.[39] In the 1990s, despite years of research, the hormonal linkage to risk-taking remained unproven.[40] Culture, or nurture versus nature, influences adolescence more than hormones.

George Stanley Hall, the American psychologist who first coined the term adolescence, wrote his influential two-volume book, *Adolescence - Its Psychology and Its Relations to Physiology, Anthropology, Sociology, Sex, Crime, and Religion*, attempting to explain adolescence as a period marked by storm and stress caused by the biological changes that came with puberty.[41] What we now call sex hormones had not yet been discovered in 1904. Hall's theory was influenced by Sigmund Freud's view that latent libido influenced all behavior during puberty.[42]

Margaret Mead published *Coming of Age in Samoa* in 1928 primarily to disprove Hall's theory of adolescence.[43] Her anthropological study demonstrated that adolescent behavior was driven by culture and society.

Studies focusing on mood and behavior changes ranging from pre-pubertal to post-pubertal young people from the 5th to the 9th grade have proven that while mood and behavior are seen to change during this time, hormone fluctuation was not positively correlated with moodiness and depression.[44] The conclusion was that environment and family status were critical to behavioral changes during these years.

The storm and stress that had traditionally been linked to biology and hormones, which made puberty and adolescence something that had to be treated medically, resulted from the environment.

Studies on the cause of risk-taking moved from hormonal development to cognitive neuroplasticity. Researchers used brain imaging the cognitive development of adolescents and concluded that the logical reasoning and mental processing ability of a 16-year-old is the same as that of an adult.[45] The storm, stress, and raging hormones our society associates with puberty and adolescence is a creation that originated in the anxieties of 19th-century society.

It was during the 19th century that society became obsessed with a post-pubertal girl's sexuality. The entirety of the Victorian response to puberty was built on a fear of sex. However, Margaret Mead's *Coming of Age in Samoa* and research into hunter-gatherer societies illustrate that earlier sexual activity did not cause early childbearing. The concern and the health issues about puberty and adolescence result from a novel human evolution that did not exist before agriculture. This explains the origin of the perils associated with puberty.

Today's medical interpretation of the perils of puberty morphs with the problems of adolescence. The physical and hormonal changes that bring about sexual maturation are linked to the emotional and psychosocial changes that together create the supposed perils of puberty. The impression our society has of the pubertal and adolescent female is that the physical and hormonal changes will cause not only the physical problems associated with puberty, such as menstrual issues, skin issues, and weight issues, but also emotional and psychological issues, such as self-consciousness, embarrassment, inability to handle changes, increased sexuality, which is seen as dangerous, aggressive, depressive, and volatile behavior.

Whereas the menopausal woman is told her hormones peter out and die, the young female is told she will be subject to raging hormones that are beyond her control and which will influence her body, her mind, and her behavior. This, of course, means they will need medical help to survive this period in their lives to reach the beach of adulthood safely.

Adolescence as a field of medical science is also new. Doctors used to treat humans—males, females, adults, and children as the same physiological entity. It was not until medicine became specialized in the 19th century that gynecology, pediatrics, and psychology were born. Before this time, children were treated as adults but given smaller doses. Children were seen as miniature versions of adults until this time. Pediatricians who wanted to distance themselves from other physicians did this by creating alternatives to breastmilk.[46] They claimed they had specific knowledge and skills to treat children that general practitioners did not medically.[47] With this came the instructions on infant feeding, which human females had perfected over 200,000 years ago.[48]

Pediatricians had difficulty convincing the public that children needed a doctor, different from a general practitioner. World War II brought increasing specialization to the medical sphere. In 1914, there were only 138 physicians who called themselves pediatricians. In the 1950s, this number had increased to more than 4,000.[49] But their professional worries were not over. New medical discoveries sent people to specialists instead of pediatricians. Another problem for them was that general practitioners were becoming more competitive with pediatricians for patients because they were losing patients to specialists.

For this reason, they formed the American Academy of General Practitioners (AAGP) to promote themselves as family physicians. The AAGP started training general practitioners in pediatrics. To raise their professional status, pediatricians became pediatric specialists and began incorporating new technology to offer pediatric surgery, radiology, oncology, cardiology, and endocrinology. In response, a segment of pediatricians decried specialization and subspecialization.[50]

It began using terms such as comprehensive pediatrics, developmental pediatrics, psychosocial pediatrics, and behavioral pediatrics to explain the care they offered to treat the whole patient and not an individual organ or disease. General pediatricians argued they were the best trained to treat psychology, school behavior and performance, and social behavior in children. It was not until the 1950s that adolescent medicine emerged, primarily for doctors to garner a specific population segment. The first *Handbook of Adolescent Psychology* was published in 1980, although no disease that adolescents suffered from existed that adults did not suffer from.[51]

Before adolescence, there was just youth. Youth could range from 7 to 30, had more to do with culture and economic class, and was more an indication of the person's financial dependence on their parents. Since the advent of agriculture, high birth rates made child labor unessential. Children were sent away to work for relatives. Boys became apprentices, but girls worked in households until they could be married.

My grandmother experienced indentured servitude. My great-grandmother died not long after she gave birth to my grandmother. Her father remarried and sent her away from Boatland, Tennessee, to live with a family in Donelson. She cared for the other children and cleaned the house until she went to school to become a teacher.

The word adolescence was first used in the 15th century to describe growing into maturity. Aristotle had written about stages in boys' lives—infancy, boyhood, and young manhood that became before adulthood, but this was only applied to males. The first work to address adolescence as a separate stage in life was George Stanley Hall's. Hall coined the term adolescence and described it as a period ranging from 14 to 24. The storm and stress he wrote that endangered the adolescent was a direct translation of the 18th century musical and literary period that expressed emotional turmoil and extreme passion. His book was an attempt to "directly and indirectly help the young to exploit aright all the possibilities of the years from fourteen to twenty-four and to safeguard them against the above insidious dangers."[52]

Hall's huge two volumes addressed everything from physical growth and health to hygiene, productivity, and moral behavior. He was addressing boys (he wrote little about females, as he thought that girls needed to stay home and become wives and mothers) after puberty.

Hall's theory of adolescence evolved from the anxiety in 19th century England and the United States about the emerging youth class created after the Industrial Revolution. Not much was changed in agricultural communities. The Industrial Revolution created cities, and with cities came the middle class and more freedom and activities for young people.

Beginning in the mid-19th century, middle-class children started going to school. The middle-class child suddenly had more freedom. This freedom caused a great deal of hand-wringing in all professional literature. A distinction was made between the home and the workplace. Before the Industrial Revolution, the home was the house you slept in. In the 19th century, the home became the hearth, and the outside world was considered dangerous.[53] Young people being led astray became a fixation for society. An example would be how masturbation became viewed as depravity when, before this time, it was something that was taken for granted and not connected to morality.[54]

Puberty became sexualized, and society became obsessed with this potential sexuality. Puberty, previously greeted by ceremonial rites of passage in most cultures, became a time that could cause danger. Writers during this period pointed out dangers and temptations threatening young people who went through puberty in urban areas. This danger was possible in boys, but since boys don't get pregnant, the worries focused more on girls. Society was concerned about the proper development of boys, but for girls, the fear became oppressive and more controlling.[55]

The Boy Scout movement was founded at this time by Baden Powell as a means to protect and foster masculinity in boys.[56] Doctors recommended and sold anti-masturbation corsets, spiky urethral rings, and metal penis caps to prevent boys from getting erections, to prevent spermatorrhoea,[57] a newly invented disease caused by both masturbation and nocturnal emissions due to the belief that boys would be weakened and possibly become insane if they lost precious sperm.

Still, a girl's virtue and future ability to fulfill her role as wife and mother were foremost on parents' minds. Doctors, theologians, and legislators took advantage of these fears and developed theories of the physical and mental frailty of the female girl, which is the source of how puberty and adolescence are viewed today.

From the mid-19th century to the end of it, puberty had been the focus of most medical treatises.[58] Hall drove the preoccupation with the period that went from puberty to the end of physical growth, what we now call the teen years. He made the divide between boy and girl even wider. He rescued boys from school work and responsibilities but drove the girl deeper into the home. Hall recommended sports, outdoor activities, and a return to childhood activities to ensure the adolescent boy became a virile man. Girls, on the other hand, had to suspend schooling, stay home and crochet, or their ability to bear children would be endangered.

The fear of childhood sexuality evolved during this time. Freud's theory of childhood sexuality was formed from Victorian society's anxiety about the potential for sexual corruption that came with the new freedoms young people had after the Industrial Revolution. Even though birth rates declined during this period, to the point of crisis during the Anglo-Boer War in 1899, when England could not recruit enough soldiers from the upper classes (the poor were too malnourished and unhealthy to make good soldiers) to fight in South Africa due to the lower birth rate, the young person's body became something that needed to be controlled and regulated.[59] Female sexuality was more dangerous than male sexuality, to the point that its existence became questioned for the first time. This period gave birth to the weak, manic, anxious, depressed, irresponsible, and hysterical adolescent girl.

Puberty and adolescence for the modern girl have not changed much from the British, Victorian, and American Gilded Age eras. Now, as then, countless books, magazines, and movies address this period in a girl's life as if it had been a fact of life throughout history, even though adolescence has only existed for a little over 100 years.[60] Modern medical theory does not question the idea that puberty and adolescence are "perilous" to the physical and mental health of a girl. Medicine blames sex hormones for behavioral and psychological issues such as anxiety, depression, and the much-bandied "risk-taking" associated with girls during their teen years.[61]

The change in diet caused menarche to come at an earlier age. Humans evolved into a species with a large brain on a diet of meat and animal fat. The invention of agriculture was a response to the scarcity of animals to hunt when they stopped being nomadic. The addition of carbohydrates to the human diet sped up female development.[62] This is indeed caused by hormones, but it is a hormonal imbalance, not the fault of the hormones themselves. Humans evolved to mature more slowly than other primates.[63] We grow up more slowly, have fewer babies, larger brains, larger bodies, longer gestation, later weaning, and live longer than other primates. Humans evolved altricial (meaning born helpless) to accommodate the larger brain that evolved with the animal protein and fat diet. The more helpless an animal is born, the larger is its brain. Compared to other primates, humans are born altricial. Our larger brain is the reason we are born helpless.[64]

Puberty, which is physiologically timed to come at the same time as a pubertal growth spurt, is now coming much sooner than it did to prehistoric girls. Females are supposed to mature later to ensure they have the physical capacity to give birth and the mental capacity to be mothers. This change in diet intensified after the Industrial Revolution. The combination of stress, changing social mores, and malnourishment are the causes of the health issues associated with puberty and adolescence.

Medications for these issues not caused by anything physiological are not the answer. Medications have side effects. Any tinkering with the endocrine system will change the secretion rate of other hormones. You can think of the endocrine system as a giant web. If you pull any strand at any part of the web, you will change the shape of the entire web. That is what medicines do. Medicines are needed to treat acute physiological deficiencies, as in the case of someone with an adrenal tumor, which prevents the normal secretion of hormones vital to existence. They should not be used to treat imbalances. They create more imbalance and will impact a girl's entire life.

TWO

A HISTORY OF THE HEALTH ISSUES OF PUBERTAL AND ADOLESCENT GIRLS

THE MODERN IDEA OF WHAT an adolescent girl is and what causes her health issues in the Western world is based on flawed concepts that developed during the 19th century, specifically the Victorian era in Britain and the Gilded Age in the United States. These two periods in history gave birth to the modern girl.[1] This is also the period during which medical professionals consolidated their professional and social status and became judges of moral control over females and their sexuality.[2]

Until the 19th century, children were miniature versions of adults. In the Middle Ages, childhood did not exist.[3] Sociologist Jeffrey Weeks wrote that they were exposed to "social aspects of adult sexuality earlier than modern children" and thus "probably had much less difficulty in coping with their biological changes."[4] The later age of puberty and menstruation of 17 also helped. Before the Industrial Revolution, youth lasted from the first signs of independence in a child to marriage. There was no adolescence.

The Industrial Revolution created cities. Young people moved from farms where boys helped their parents or became apprentices, a form of indentured servitude. The boys sent money to their parents, who had paid a large sum to gain them an apprenticeship.

Girls were mini-moms. They helped their mothers with housekeeping, farm chores, and younger children. The factories that the Industrial Revolution created needed young workers, and girls got jobs in the cities for the first time. Despite the chances for education, the beginning of the suffrage movement to get women the right to vote, and some murmuring from physicians that married women should have fewer children for health reasons and more access to birth control, this was not a time of liberation.[5]

Social and medical views on sexuality changed. The 18th century brought a massive change in how women were viewed by society. Before the Age of Enlightenment, a period extending from roughly 1685 to 1815, women were considered the same sex as men, only inferior, due to menstruation making them cold and moist. They could not burn toxins as well as men. This was the only difference between the male and female body. Galen, the Roman Greek physician, described the different reproductive organs as inverted versions of male organs. Referencing the record of dissections by the Alexandrian anatomist, Herophilus, Galen listed the vagina as an internal version of the penis, the labia as the foreskin, the uterus as the scrotum, and the ovaries were the testicles.[6]

For two millennia, the ovaries were called by the same Greek word for testicles, orcheis. Similar to a man's need to orgasm to release sperm, there was also a belief that a woman having intercourse without orgasm would not lead to pregnancy. Men and women could turn into the other. The literature described men who lactated and girls who became boys.

A 16th century physician wrote how a girl suddenly grew a penis and a scrotum. A modern medical explanation would say she perhaps had adrenal hyperplasia and developed both male and female genitalia and that the testicles descended when she was chasing the pigs, as described in the account. Still, the idea was not unscientific at the time. Ursula Le Guin's novel, *The Left Hand of Darkness*, describes the Gethenians as having no fixed gender. The inhabitants of the planet Gethen had a 26-day cycle where they were androgynous, after which came a 2-3 day cycle during which they were sexually active as either male or female, having no control over which gender the cycle would choose.[7] This and Virginia Woolf's novel about the nobleman Orlando, who turns into a woman after a stressful event after spending two centuries as a male, would have seemed less fantastical to scientists pre-Enlightenment.[8]

In the late 18th century, the idea of human sexuality changed. Medical literature argued the ancient physicians had been wrong. Women were completely different from men in every possible way. They were weak and passive, while men were strong and energetic. Many books were published in German, French, and English about how the female body and her morality differed from the male's. They used this new interpretation of the female sex to explain the cultural, political, and economic differences between women's and men's status in society. Even the existence of female sexual pleasure disappeared.[9] Medical writers jumped into the fray with new theories about the perils of puberty and female biological limitations. Whereas previously, a woman was simply a failed man. Medicine believed that female physiology was an upside down and flawed version of the male. It wasn't until the 18th century that two different genders became accepted.

Nothing scientific had happened to cause this change from one sex to two sexes. Hormones had not been discovered. Ovulation was still a mystery to physicians, but somehow, the facts changed. Anatomical evidence proved that all humans start out as the same gender in the womb when scientists discovered that embryologically the penis, the clitoris, the labia, the scrotum, the ovaries, and the testes originated from the same fetal tissue.[10]

Why the change in thinking? There were enormous cultural and economic shifts happening. The French Revolution had frightened the aristocracy and gave birth to post-revolution conservatism. There was a rise in evangelical religion. The free market economy and industrialization were born, bringing stark class differences and a sexual division of labor.

Some 50 years later, in Victorian England and 70 years later in the United States, during the so-called Gilded Age, reform movements tried to temper the changes in the lives of adolescents. The temperance, hygienic health, protestant Adventist, vegetarian, and spiritualism movements all appealed to new Victorian morality and national and social identity.[11]

Influential Victorians became involved with dietary change as a means of addressing not only health but also morality. The Vegetarian Society was formed in Manchester in 1847 and was the first in the Western world. Several similar organizations sprung up during this period, and in 1899, the Vegetarian Society had over six thousand members.[12]

The Victorian vegetarians were influenced by the American Grahamists, and from the beginning, they were connected to the international elite of temperance and other reform movements. Popular religious and health movements began equating eating meat with sexual desire. Grahamism, a religious dietary reform movement founded by Sylvester Graham, a minister who preached that "carnal desire" caused headaches, epilepsy, and insanity.[13] Graham invented the Graham Cracker, which he designed to be brittle, tasteless, flavorless, and hard to chew. He first produced this unleavened whole wheat flour, wheat bran, and wheat germ cracker in 1829, believing it would suppress sexual desire in adolescent boys.[14] Nabisco bought it in 1890 and added the sugar and cinnamon Sylvester Graham thought would incite the sexual desire to make it the sweet snack cracker we know today.[15]

Adventism, a branch of evangelical Protestant Christianity, was founded in 1863 in the United States by Ellen G. White, who established the church based on her visions.[16] She believed that eating meat was sinful and that eating animal products would cause people to have animal desires. Members of this church founded processed food companies and have today become substantial global conglomerates that fund and push their religious ideology of a plant-based diet on the rest of us through dietary guidelines, shoddy research, and publicity campaigns.[17]

Sylvester Graham influenced the Seventh-Day Adventist co-founder Ellen G. White, whose religious visions informed her evangelical theology despite regularly eating meat venison, oysters, butter, fish, condiments, and spices,[18] all substances her visions had told her were unclean and harmful to the soul.[19]

John Harvey Kellogg, of Kellogg's cereals, was raised in the Seventh-day Adventist Church from childhood. Kellogg was selected as a protégé of Ellen G. White and trained as a doctor.[20] However, he disapproved of Whites' regularly asking the vegetarian Battle Creek Sanitarium cook to prepare her fried chicken when she visited.[21] He held a prominent role as a speaker at church meetings but also considered himself a Grahamite, and created cornflakes and granola in 1878 as a plain tasting, uninspiring food that would keep people's minds off of sex and masturbation, as he believed that sex and masturbation were not only immoral but unhealthy. He believed that it damaged the mind, caused acne, lousy posture, palpitations, and epilepsy and that foods such as meat and butter caused people to have the carnal desire, and nuts and cereals suppressed it. He opened the Battle Creek Sanitarium as a health resort in Michigan in 1866, based on the health principles published by Ellen G. Whites's visions of removing meat, butter, sugar, and alcohol from the diet.[22]

"Kellogg was more responsible than any other person in his generation for popularizing the fallacious disease of masturbation," author John Money wrote in his book, The *Destroying Angel: Sex, Fitness, and Food in the Legacy of Degeneracy Theory, Graham Crackers, Kellogg s Corn Flakes, and American Health History.*[23]

He and his brother, Will Keith Kellogg, founded the Battle Creek Sanitarium Health Food Company in 1898 to produce food stuffs for current and former patients at Dr. J.H. Kellogg's sanitarium, the Battle Creek Sanitarium. The company later became known as the Battle Creek Sanitarium Food Company in 1901. They also sold nut butter and other meat substitutes. The company merged with the Sanitas Nut Food Company, founded in 1899 by Kellogg.[24] Kellogg is one of the largest and most influential companies today, consistently claiming to promote health with its sugary, processed products. Dr. J.H. Kellogg not only invented the breakfast cereal, but he also conducted 22,000 surgeries.[25] His treatment for young women caught masturbating was either the chemical desensitizing of the clitoris or removing it entirely.[26]

Maximilian Oskar Bircher-Benner, a Swiss doctor who also founded a sanitarium, invented Muesli for the same reasons in 1900 but used oats and added apples instead of cornflakes.[27] Still, the idea was the same—an anti-meat agenda promoted for religious reasons marketed as health care.

In Germany and Switzerland, the Lebensreform movement espoused the vegetarian diet and naturopathy in response to urbanization from the Industrial Revolution.[28] Sebastian Kneipp, a Catholic priest famous for hydrotherapy, was one of the originators of the Nature

Cure and Kneipp societies that later became known as naturopathic societies.[29] Both Kneipp and Rudolf Steiner, a famous educator who founded Steiner Education, were prominent members of the Lebensreform movement.[30]

Many women were attracted to these movements. Women were associated with diet and family morality, and men were happy to have them in leadership roles.[31] Food and diet became a way for the upper and middle classes to differentiate themselves from the lower classes and foreigners. The evangelical protestants equated eating meat with the sins of sensuality and gluttony. Until this time, corpulence had been associated with health, but this changed, and eating beyond satiation was seen as debauchery. The health and evangelical reform movements exploited the upper and middle-class fears of the pathology of urban and industrial living. A reformed diet that eliminated meat was promoted as a form of self-control and self-restraint that led to more spiritual behavior.

The elite in Western societies were terrified of overpopulation. This fear had been instilled by the British economist Thomas Malthus' *Essay on the Principle of Population*. British society was gripped by a Malthusian anxiety of overbreeding by the poor after the India Mutiny in 1857.[32] The upper classes were afraid of being overrun by the poor. Britain and other colonial powers were afraid of being overrun by the natives, and the United States was afraid of being overrun by immigrants. The Irish potato famine in the mid-19th century brought nearly one million Irish immigrants to New York.[33] The socio-political changes that followed the Italian War of Unification in 1848 brought over two million southern Italian immigrants to New York's shores.[34]

In the mid-1800s, industrialization caused a migration of people from the countryside in England and the United States to the urban areas around factories,[35] and in Britain's case, an influx of people from the colonies as the British empire crumbled.[36] This created a population explosion in the cities. A middle class was born when, before, the only classes had been the aristocracy, the artisans, and the peasantry.

Instead of the overpopulation Thomas Malthus warned of, the opposite came to pass. When Britain tried to recruit male soldiers to fight in the Anglo-Boer war in 1899, it found that volunteers from lower classes weren't healthy enough to be recruited, and the lower birth rate in the upper classes meant there weren't enough men to send to war.[37] This caused consternation and the assumption that women were focused on education, employment, and the new idea of emancipation rather than having children. We see this anxiety resonating in the propaganda of right-wing movements in Europe today in countries where the fear of immigration and a continued alarm that the women of the nationality associated with the country of the movement do not have enough children to equal the birth rate of immigrants. The erosion of women's rights today is a direct consequence of this thinking, as it was in the 19th century.

Urban societies created a new woman. She went to school. She read novels and newspapers. The Romantic literary movement also impacted women's food choices. The famous poet Percy Shelley wrote that eating meat was the "root of all evil."[38] He was a vegetarian, as was his wife, Mary Shelley, who wrote *Frankenstein*. Lord Byron, the most famous poet of the Victorian era, was also a vegetarian.

The new woman was scary enough, but the new young woman was even more frightening. The new girl frightened social commentators. Society feared the docile feminine ideal created in the 18th century during the Age of Enlightenment would be lost. Medical theories became based on these ideals. Girls were considered biologically unstable and physiologically weaker than boys because of their reproductive organs.[39] The new girl who worked in factories became seen as potentially deviant because she was not at home with her parents. The upper and middle-class girl who went to school, read books, and went to parties was exposed to realities it was thought she would not be able to handle, let alone defend her virtue from.[40] Life for girls became more complex.

This period is when girls became two kinds of people—the depraved girl who ignored social mores and only thought about sex and the docile, asexual good girl.[41] Sexuality was no longer supposed to exist for her. The pubertal girl was a danger to society and herself if she did not conform to the new gendered idea of the asexual female.

Middle-class girls started going to school, which they had never done before. Boys were traditionally educated. Girls were not. Upper and middle-class girls went to school to differentiate themselves from the uneducated factory and farm girls. Without farm chores, these girls now had more time on their hands. They not only went to school, but they also learned to play instruments and went to dances. Medical men, and they were still only men until the late 19th century, argued that the pursuit of education or emancipation would endanger their mental and physical health. They wrote that the sole activity girls were born to, their ability to be wives and produce children, would be endangered.[42]

The greater independence young people had access to in cities created a fervor of fear in the upper classes. This fear made its way into the medical and social discourse of the time. During the nineteenth century, women's health, previously the purview of midwives, came under the control of the new medical specialties of obstetrics, gynecology, and psychology. Women were barred from medical schools in all countries until the end of the 19th century. The medical world saw a woman's reproductive system as the source of all female diseases and health issues. Hippocrates believed that the uterus could wander through a woman's body and cause anxiety, toxins, and even paralysis. His cure for ill women was marriage and sex to prevent the uterus from wandering. Roman Aulus Cornelius Celsus wrote that the womb caused epilepsy. Galen's take was that the uterus caused anxiety and that women with what has been called hysteria since Hippocrates named it a female disease had to be treated with laudanum, belladonna, and valerian root, much like how anxiety is treated today, benzodiazepines, and anti-depressants, all derived from toxic plants.[43]

Young women were viewed as either sinners or victims, and their sexuality had to be controlled by the family, the church, schools, and, increasingly, the state.[44] However, no professional entity wanted to claim responsibility for female adolescent sexuality. Their sexuality needed to be controlled, and strategies for control gave rise to, as Nathanson writes, "the medical profession as a center of cultural authority over the management of social problems and to changes in socially acceptable roles for women" in *Dangerous Passage: The Social Control of Sexuality in Women's Adolescence.*[45] Since the 19th century, sexuality has become the primary cause of social disorder.

With pregnancy, a female adolescent's sexuality becomes visible in a way that will never happen with a male. Before the 19th century, girls grew up to get married. With the Industrial Revolution, more middle-class families educated their daughters, and jobs became available. These changes culminated with the suffragette movement born in East London in 1907 and climaxed with the women's vote in 1918 in the United Kingdom and 1920 in the United States. Italy and New Zealand serve as two bookends—women in New Zealand gained the right to vote in 1893, yet Italian women didn't get the right to vote until 1945. Society has been wringing its hands about female adolescent sexuality since the 1800s and has sought to contain it. Cultural ideas about female sexuality were formed by the concept that sexuality is uncontrollable and a biological force; thus, for women, the time between puberty and marriage had to be asexual.

Girls were sent to homes for "wayward girls," psychiatric institutions, birth control clinics, and maternity homes.[46] From the mid-1900s, unwed pregnant girls were sent to church "mother and baby" homes in Ireland run by Catholic Churches. Investigation into these types of homes from 1922 to 1998 uncovered that illegal vaccine trials, abuse, and horrible living conditions caused the death of 9000 mothers and the babies that were taken away from them.[47] The issue has always been unwanted pregnancy. Even though the medical establishment has taken on the management of female sexuality and the control of "deviance," diseases can be treated and cured, but sexuality cannot.

The surgeons of the 19th century did not stop there. Since a woman's female organs were the cause of all her ailments, and since it was reasoned she only needed those to have babies, surgeons treated hysteria, melancholy, nymphomania, and insanity by removing the ovaries.[48] A woman was often labeled insane if she did not conform to the rigid confines of social norms and conventions. More women than men ended up in insane asylums.[49] Fathers, brothers, and husbands often committed women.[50] A study of admissions records of women admitted to an asylum in the United States from 1860-1900 lists the reasons for admissions as insane by menses, insane by religious excitement, insane by overwork and domestic trouble, insane by childbirth, insane by nymphomania, and insane by suppressed menses.[51] Records showed that admitted women had attacks of insanity one to two weeks a month that correlated with their cycle.[52]

Medical historian Thomas Schlich wrote that the 19th century was a "crucial stage in the history of modern surgery."[53] An ensemble of new technologies led to a new style of surgery and facilitated an unprecedented extension of the range and number of surgical interventions. Surgeons were eager to try out their new techniques on women. Women have been historically experimented on more than men. Unfortunately, this has been on minority women and women in insane asylums and institutions and had no control over what was happening to them.

Since post-pubertal girls menstruated, they were seen as invalids during their cycle. All diseases that women had were related to their reproductive organs. Puberty, physicians argued, was particularly dangerous. Medical literature did not focus this concern on boys. Females were seen as having a limited amount of energy. If a girl spent this energy on educating herself or participating in activities, she would be spent before she married and was expected to have children. The fact that girls bled, losing a substance monthly, seemed to support this belief that post-pubertal girls were losing some of their vitality monthly. It was not understood until decades later that menstruating was a shedding endometrium and served a healthy purpose as part of a healthy female cycle.

Girls were considered to be prone to disease, disorders, and deviance. They had to be sequestered to reduce danger to them. Ill health, which until this time had been considered dependent upon the constitution of the individual, became the concern of both British and American psyches because it could be caused by immorality. The female adolescent's health would decide the white race's well-being. The new medical field of psychology contributed to this view. In an attempt to advance their careers in their specialty, obstetrical surgeons argued the origin of the girls' illnesses was pathological, and psychiatrists argued the origin of the girls' illnesses was psychological.

Most of the concern focused on middle-class girls. Organizations such as the YWCA and others were created to focus on the factory girls, but concerns about girls of the upper classes dominated literature. The malnourishment described by Charles Dickens in *A Christmas Story* was common in mid-19th century cities in England. There were food reform movements at this time that tried to address the malnourishment of the poor. The United States was seen as a wealthy cousin that did not suffer the food scarcity that the English working class did at this time.[54] By the end of the 19th century, nutritional benefits to working girls became a consideration as well. Still, this class of girls was not diagnosed with the variety of illnesses that seemed to plague upper and middle-class girls. Their sexuality did, however, need to be controlled.

During this period, society became obsessed with controlling sex. Physicians, psychiatrists, physicians, lawyers, judges, and educators became involved in making rules about sex and sexuality. In 1860, the British parliament passed the Contagious Diseases Act that forced working-class women suspected of prostitution to undergo medical examinations.[55] Men who were their customers were never subjected to this treatment. During this period, pornography, a word first used in 1864, also evolved into the form familiar to us today, allowing upper-class males to indulge in fantasies involving lower-class women.[56] The concept of eugenics evolved from the fear of girls from higher classes choosing education and emancipation over their biological duty to continue with the white race.[57]

Surgery as a means of addressing a girl's health issues became commonplace and widespread during the middle part of the 19th century. Oophorectomy was commonly referred to as Battey's Operation, for the American gynecologist who performed hundreds of them to treat menstrual disorders, epilepsy, and mania.[58] Critics of Robert Battey at the time wondered if surgeons were inventing disorders to cure them in a surge of commercialism that was rampant in medicine. Masturbation, which became an obsession in Victorian and American society at this time, was treated by clitoridectomy.

A London gynecologist, Lawson Tait, the creator of Tait's Law, stated, "When in doubt, open the belly to find out."[59] Hundreds of women died during these surgeries. A successful British gynecologist, Isaac Baker Brown, published a book about treating masturbation, which he claimed was caused by the hypertrophy and irritation of the clitoris. This supposed hypertrophy would, according to him, interfere with fertility, and the only solution was clitoris removal. Hypertrophy of the clitoris sounds a lot like modern plastic surgeons treating what they call hypertrophic labia minora with labiaplasty. Brown's second book, *The Curability of Certain Forms of Insanity, Epilepsy, and Hysteria in Females*, was published in 1866. Thankfully, he was finally forced to close his clinic because he got in trouble, not for maiming women but for not having consulted with the husbands of the women he operated on.[60] He died bankrupt.

The controversy of clitoridectomy discussed in several medical journals underlined how many doctors during this period viewed female sexuality as dangerous and menacing when it was not in the confines of reproduction during marriage. Clitorectomy fell out of favor in the United Kingdom at the turn of the century but continued to be performed in the United States until the 1950s.[61]

Social commentators feared the modern girl who wanted to go to school, get a job, and not simply stay home and raise a family. These unfeminine characteristics seemed dangerous.

Feminine characteristics were sharply aligned with the new docile, weak, and waif-like female whose only purpose was to please her husband, give birth to children, and manage the home. The robust women who worked on farms were associated with the lower classes.

There was massive anxiety about sexuality, gender, and morality, which included ideology, science, medicine, and legal practices. The domestic hearth became crucial to uphold morality and social mores. The definitions of femininity and masculinity became sharply divided.

This was when sports became included in educational institutions for the first time. Organizations like the Boy Scouts were created to ensure boys became masculine enough, starkly dichotomizing the gender differences between boys and girls in a new way.[62] Professional sports teams were formed, which guided boys towards masculinity and gave them males to root for. The ideal boy was strong and vigorous, with elements of brutality necessary to go to war.

The ideal female, on the other hand, was docile, weak, and only interested in homemaking. Doctors noted that girls who lived in cities started menstruating earlier than farm girls. Urban life was too stimulating for the weak nervous system of girls, so they needed extra protection. Girls who had climbed trees with their brothers had to be kept inside as soon as they reached puberty to ready them for the strain of menstruation. Girls had to be guided into womanhood for the benefit of the nation. Parents were warned that too much exercise and study would weaken their ability to have children later and possibly cause not only infertility, hysteria, and irrationality but also insanity. The onset of puberty, seen as the cause of emotional upheaval and instability, was the biggest threat to the young female mind.

Most medical literature of this time cautioned that higher education and exercise were dangerous to young women.[63] Medical literature raised the alarm that activities outside the home, and even schooling inside the home, would cause them nervous distress and illnesses. Mothers were advised that their daughters had to be kept home in tranquility to fulfill their purpose as mothers. Educating their daughters would create infertile, pale, flat-chested, boyish girls.[64] All professions shared the medical writers' concerns, including legislators, school headmistresses, girls' club directors, gymnastics teachers, and journalists. As Michel Foucault asserted in *The History of Sexuality*, science drove a discussion about the human body to bring it under the control and power of a wide range of professions in a way that wasn't seen before.[65]

Medical professionals presented images of young girls as susceptible to mental and physical degeneration. The weak girl could also become the frighteningly erotic girl, who, if allowed to engage in masturbation, would be plagued by morbid impulses, fatigue, and depression—all symptoms of girls who were diagnosed with the illnesses associated with puberty. A pubertal girl's weak nervous system made her particularly predisposed to nymphomania and sexual delusions.[66]

How girls dressed was seen to contribute to their health issues. The female body was fetishized to heighten the physical difference from the male body. Corsets were tight-laced to the point of causing damage to internal organs and ribs. Various professionals, from physicians to preachers, criticized corsets as not only dangerous as they could move a girl's ribs and squeeze her reproductive organs in a way that was dangerous to her fertility but also evidence of the frivolousness and immorality of middle-class and aristocratic girls' obsession with their appearance.[67] Reform movements evolving at the time, such as the emancipation movement in Britain and the anti-slavery and temperance movements in the United States, initiated the importance of clothes for women that did not restrict their movement and spoke of the corsets as being part of the patriarchal desire to keep women subservient to men. The feminine ideal would change from exaggerated curves to the androgynous shape of the flapper soon after World War I.

Since girls had a growth spurt before boys, they were seen as developing dangerously faster than them. Tall girls were seen as unfeminine, but this "deformity" could not be treated until the discovery of hormones and the subsequent marketing of them. Treating the unfeminine stature of tall girls with estrogen would not begin until the 1940s.[68] But Victorian mothers would probably have rushed their daughters to physicians if such treatment had been available. Studies about the medicalization of tall girls showed that it was mothers concerned about the attractiveness of their daughters who initiated the treatment of girls as young as eight. Until the invention of synthetic hormones, the cultural ideals of femininity rooted in medical practices took the form of advice to parents on how to sequester their daughters, calming drugs, surgery, and psychoanalysis.

Pathological conditions were discovered. Hysteria had always been associated with women, but physicians treated newer pathologies associated with the female reproductive system. There was an explosion in medical literature dedicated to the illnesses that endangered female adolescents.

Four diseases came to be associated with adolescence—hysteria, neurasthenia, anorexia nervosa, and chlorosis. Chlorosis has disappeared as a diagnosis, replaced by different forms of anemia, but anorexia nervosa and hysteria, although called by different names, are still health issues associated with adolescent females. Physicians wrote that girls pretended to be ill and that they used illness as a weapon against men. Their imagination was seen as a danger to themselves and the men in their lives. Freud's famous case history of his 14-year-old patient Dora, who exhibited, according to him, hysteria instead of genital stimulation when she became disgusted by the advances of her father's much older friend, is an excellent example of the medical thinking of that time.[69]

Scottish medical doctor and criminologist Sir Horatio Donkin's 1882 essay on hysteria described that adolescent girls were most likely to suffer from hysteria caused by a nervous imbalance due to changes in their sex organs.[70] He wrote that the young female, who had less nervous resiliency than the male, would thus suffer more imbalance during puberty. He also seemed to empathize with the fact that girls were controlled and prevented from education and ignorance about sexuality. He wrote that the relative freedom boys had offered them an outlet for their nervous tensions. While working-class adolescents went to work, middle-class and aristocratic girls were groomed for marriage while watching their brothers go to school and engage in activities. Donkin reiterated Hippocrates' theory that unsatisfied sexual desire caused hysteria.[71] The absence of stimulation and activity was harmful, but so were the studying and exercise. What was a girl to do?

Neurasthenia was an advanced form of hysteria that plagued more upper-class girls and women. Its symptoms were lack of energy, appetite, and low concentration. George Beard, a doctor in Boston, named the disease in 1869 as a form of nervous exhaustion and blamed its rampant spread through upper-class girls on urbanization and industrialization that came after the Civil War. J.G. Biller, MD of Iowa, wrote in 1902 that "I have seen these delicate women—that unfortunate class who are launched into life with a nervous system so frail that it can scarcely supply sufficient nerve force to meet the ordinary demands of living—I have seen these delicate women systematically starved for years, while they underwent all kinds of scientific treatment: drugs galore, electricity, massage and even starvation by rule at well-known sanitariums." Dr. Biller advocated "a liberal diet of common-sense food" and not "a diet of high-priced concentrated food."[72]

In 1873, Sir William Withey Gull, one of Queen Victoria's personal physicians, published a paper about a condition that afflicted young women he called Anorexia Nervosa. That same year, Ernest-Charles Lasègue, a French neurologist, published a paper called De l'Anorexie Hystérique, with the word hysteria immediately associated with females.[73] Girls stopped eating. It was middle-class primarily and upper-class girls who stopped eating in the 1870s. Anorexia Nervosa was considered to be caused by anxiety about schoolwork. Many doctors wrote that girls were faking it.

There has been a long history of girls not eating, well-illustrated in Joan Jacobs Brumberg's book *Fasting Girls: The History of Anorexia Nervosa*. In the Middle Ages, there had been instances of girls gripped by religious fervor who claimed to survive solely on the eucharist—wafers and wine—given to them during church services. Brumberg demonstrates extensively the medieval scholarship that recounted many girls who refused to eat. The ability to refuse or limit food during those times was associated with purity and divinity.[74] That a human could subsist only their faith may have been attractive to young women who had no outlet other than becoming wives and having children.

The fact that many girls refused to eat during the Middle Ages signifies that the disease was not born during the Victorian era. Still, it also underlines how not only a young female's limited choices can be a driver to refuse food to get some control over their life but also how denial of food, always associated with fleshly pursuits by religion, is associated with asceticism.

Increased asceticism was part of the reform movements' goals that influenced culture at this time. The temperance, spiritualism, and evangelical protestant movements warned against the sin and debauchery that society was doomed to be engulfed in after the Industrial Revolution. Upper and middle-class girls, in their new role as keepers of virtue in the home, could not escape the increased pressure to fulfill the image of femininity that society thrust upon them. This also meant denying fleshly necessities like eating. The longer these girls fasted, the more people were convinced of their purity and saint-like ability to exist without food. Catherine of Siena, the 14th century Italian theologian canonized 80 years after her death by starvation, demonstrated her piety not only by fasting but also by flagellating herself, burning her skin, and cutting herself. I will explain in a later chapter how stress hormones produced by these kinds of activities can give a kind of physiological solace that will drive a person to continue self-harm.

Anorexia has always been more prevalent in upper and middle-class society. The fact that Victorian girls of the upper and middle-class society did it, and girls who lived on farms or worked in factories did not, is not so much an indication that those with plenty chose to refuse food but more an illustration of how girls identified themselves with the changing mores of their society. Studies have shown that during times of hardship, such as war, when food was scarce, there were little to no cases of anorexia. Hilda Bruch, who has written extensively on Anorexia, wrote that "The illness used to be the accomplishment of an isolated girl who felt she had found her own way to salvation. Now, it is more a group reaction."[75]

My older daughter stayed several months in a community to resolve her issues with bulimia, where she was prescribed benzodiazepines and mood stabilizers. Instead, she learned new ways to induce vomiting from other patients at the rehabilitation center. The idea that girls chose not to eat as a way of exerting some control over their lives and their bodies is one that physicians of that period brought to bear in their attempts to explain Anorexia Nervosa in the 19th century.

How much women ate became part of their femininity and indicated their morality. Poor women ate as much as they could get their hands on, but in higher society, where food was plentiful, it became fashionable for women to deny themselves. The renowned novelist, poet, and journalist Mary Ann Evans, who wrote under the pen name George Eliot, said Lord Byron stated a woman should never be seen eating.[76] This reminds me of the Duchess of Windsor's comment, "You can never be too rich or too thin."

Eating was associated with low bodily functions, such as bowel movements. Even constipation became part of the feminine ideal. Girls were taught that anything more than dietary frugality would cause ugliness and endanger their ability to find a husband. The attractive female was expected to live on air. The surge of spiritualism at this time co-opted some women's refusal or inability to eat as a sign that they could achieve this. The soul was more important than the flesh, and there were numerous accounts at this time of young women who claimed to be able to survive on nothing but their faith. The evangelical reform movements promoted the idea that the soul was separated from the flesh. One physician in New York made a wager that a girl who claimed to have fasted for 14 years must have been eating something, as it was not considered scientifically possible to survive starvation. Another girl in Boston was exhibited publicly to audiences as a scientific marvel until Dr. Mary Walker, an American surgeon and abolitionist, reported she saw her eating a piece of fried potato and declared her a fraud.[77]

Romantic poet Lord Byron lived on nothing but cookies and soda water. He fought to maintain a wraith-like thinness and hated being fat. He fasted to keep his mind sharp and his soul pure. Thousands of girls followed his example. Being thin and frail became a way for the upper classes to distinguish the rich from the poor. This has not changed. We can see evidence of this on social media and in the Western ideal body shape. Other cultures considered a small amount of body fat a sign of health. Too much is a sign of ill health. Still, emaciation is the opposite extreme, and the fact that this ideal body image originated from girls' endeavoring to conform to the distorted and flawed idea of femininity created by social anxiety in the male mind, will hopefully lead modern girls to question the origin of today's beauty standards.

The one disease that had afflicted many girls of the period that vanished at the end of the 19th century was chlorosis. The word came from the pale leaves of plants grown in mineral-deficient soil. Without minerals, plants cannot produce chlorophyll. The chlorotic girl, whose skin turned slightly green, became a poster child for the Victorian adolescent. Besides a slight green tinge to the skin that was more due to paleness than it was to its greenish hue, chlorosis, also known as green sickness, caused palpitations, amenorrhea, fainting, weight loss, headaches, fatigue, and breathlessness. Boys did not suffer from chlorosis. Some doctors believed that all girls going through puberty would have a bout of chlorosis.

This disease was less complicated for physicians, as it did not seem to have psychological components, as did hysteria, neurasthenia, and anorexia. The chlorotic girl was cured with iron salts and some bed rest. We can recognize these symptoms as caused by anemia due to iron deficiency. Pharmaceutical companies and doctors benefited from a bustling market in tonics and tablets aimed at the families of girls on the verge of puberty.[78] Some patients graduated with a diagnosis of anorexia. It was relatively easy to administer iron salts but more challenging to get a girl to eat the single food richest in iron, which is meat.

Meat was the worst food a girl could eat.[79] It was made from flesh and was not a dainty food a stylish girl should eat. That it was associated with base desires of sex and masturbation, made it even more disgusting. Chlorotic girls abstained from eating meat. Doctors told their patients that meat produced heat and could stimulate not only sexual development but also sexual activity.

Dr Lucien Warner, a New York state physician who achieved fame as a traveling lecturer, spoke about how the rigid corsets, popular at the time, could dislodge women's reproductive organs, but also about how eating meat caused breast development. He designed the Coraline Health Corset that allowed women more effortless movement in 1873, which made him a millionaire. His company exists today under the name Warnaco and makes swimsuits for Victoria's Secret and Calvin Klein Underwear.[80] Avoiding meat would delay puberty.[81] The fact that chlorotic and anorexic girl lost their period proved his point.

Mid-19th-century adolescent girls liked carbohydrates in the form of cookies and potatoes. They liked pies and fruit preserves. Meat was disgusting to them. Fatty meat was the worst. If a girl were wasting away, physicians would recommend she add meat to her diet, but neither she nor her parents were happy about this.[82] Not only was meat associated with sexuality, but doctors had been telling patients for years that female digestion was as weak as her nerves were. Meat was more difficult for her to digest than pies, potatoes, fruit, and cookies.[83] It required robust digestive mechanics. In contrast, George Stanley Hall wrote that the minds of adolescent boys needed meat.

Was it a problem of the mind or the body? Physicians believed it was the female nervous system weakened by puberty that caused their diseases. That the illnesses originated in the female reproductive organs was clear to them; how should they be treated? Surgeons primarily believed girls who refused to eat were hysterical, and hysterectomies were the cure. Neurologists and the Alienists, the name for psychologists at the time, believed the health issues were mental and not physical. These doctors criticized the popularity of hysterectomies, oophorectomies, and clitoridectomies, which removed healthy organs to treat what to them were psychological issues.[84] They also pointed out that the surgeries often failed to prevent masturbation. American neurologist George Beard, who believed neurasthenia and other "perversions" such as masturbation and homosexuality were caused by the stresses of city life, railed against these surgeries and believed female hysteria and neurasthenia to be caused by disturbance to the nervous system. Beard blamed the girls' refusal to eat meat on Lord Byron and the Calvinist doctrine that equated satiety with sin.[85]

History repeats itself, but what was more black and white in the 19th century, today has many shades of grey. My mother, who fasted to get into her wedding dress in 1958 and who my 10-year-old self remembers castigating herself for eating a box of Triscuits when she was depressed, never made meat a priority. She loved baking cakes and pies more than she liked making roasts. After years of being a healthy weight until her early 30s, she spent the rest of her life so thin that when she fell, she fractured her hip in 11 places. She was diagnosed with a thyroid issue in her 50s, which would have contributed to not only her depression but also her yo-yo dieting. She looked fantastic in the designer clothes given to her when she was a journalist in Paris covering fashion week, but she also asked her husband if she'd gained weight when she had Alzheimer's in her 80s. He pointed out that the designer clothes he'd vehemently criticized her for accepting from the designers when he met her still fit.

I, in turn, resorted to a 500-calorie diet that I found in a poisonous paperback in the health section of a local bookstore at 15. That is when I got my period, and I remember fainting twice. Once after a hot shower and once on a school ski trip. My mother wholly supported my breakfast of tea and a single slice of whole wheat toast, the large glass jars of mixed raw vegetables shaken with mayonnaise I took to school for lunch, and the dinner of one single can of green beans. I became slender and fit into the same size jeans as my best friend at the time, the most popular girl in my grade, fit into.

I took a two-year hiatus from this insanity when I gave the middle finger to the establishment and hung out with the hardcore punk of Washington, DC, most of whom I went to high school with. Skinny and fashionable were irrelevant. What was important was questioning authority, not fitting in, and not looking like or buying what everyone else did. Yet, during my first year of college, I was alone and figured out how not to eat by snorting cocaine in the Columbia University bathroom during bathroom breaks. I had to pee a lot since stimulants activate the sympathetic nervous system. This was a lonely enterprise. I studied for exams and worked long shifts in restaurants. I did not party. I got pregnant at 18, had an abortion, and from thereon, my body refused to allow me to lose weight through starvation. This was because the pregnancy had triggered a biological response. No more would it let me endanger my possible progeny by damaging it through fasting. I took up running, finished school, and had children. I never thought so much about my weight after that. I ran too often, but being a mother changed my focus from my search for the "ideal weight" to nutrition. I hadn't learned enough yet. Although meat and animal protein were always a part of dinner after my children were weaned, I'm sure the peanut butter sandwiches alternating with cheese and ham weren't enough protein or cholesterol to help their ability to focus at school.

My 15-year-old older daughter gained weight after she started taking the birth control prescribed to her by a gynecologist in Italy whom I had asked to fit her for a diaphragm since I did not want her to take birth control pills. I had never used them. She and her nurse laughed at me and said the Italian National Health Service did not offer barrier methods. My insistence mortified my daughter. My still-lingering American accent probably mortified her as well. She started vomiting as a means of getting rid of the weight instead of suspending the birth control. Today, she is a healthy 35-year-old carnivore who I know will give much thought to her grandmother's, mine, and her experience if she has a daughter.

THREE

WHAT IS PUBERTY?

PUBERTY IS A SECOND BIRTH. During puberty, our endocrine system orchestrates changes in hormone levels similar to what a neonate experiences. Adolescence happens for both girls and boys. The health issues I address here actually influence a man's life in very similar ways, yet it is society and how women are viewed by it that makes it so different and challenging for girls.

While this is indeed a health book to help young women navigate the health issues that arise in adolescence, I have to explain how society affects a young woman's health. In my previous book, I demonstrated that male perception of menopause turned it into an illness, which it isn't. Science had nothing to do with it. Puberty and adolescence suffer from the same misperception. Young women are prescribed medications, and illnesses are associated with their turning from girls to young women with reproductive potential. Male perception of what adolescence means causes adolescent women to be prescribed certain medications that adolescent men are not.

Many things have changed since I was an adolescent, but so much is the same. It is still a time fraught with insecurity and changes that can cause damaging amounts of stress. How our bodies change in adolescence affects our health and how we see ourselves for the rest of our lives. I want this book to help young women avoid the pitfalls society, not their changing bodies, throws in their way so they can reach old age with all their bits and pieces and their mental and physical health intact.

Biochemically, puberty is a time of change of massive endocrine changes. These changes include both physical and mental changes. We cannot separate the brain and its function from the rest of physiology, so I will continue by describing these changes as part of one single biological change—the formation of sexual characteristics. The human brain continues to grow until a person is about 28 years old. However, sexual characteristics are formed during puberty. The second chapter explains that the creation of the idea of adolescence in society and in medicine is very new. Physiologically, it is puberty that exerts changes on the body, but it is culture and society that cause the stress that can affect both mental and physical health during adolescence.[1] Supporting this endocrine and neuroendocrine change ensures the health of the rest of a female's life. For this reason, I have chosen to use the word puberty to describe these changes.

Hundreds of female patients have told me their health issues started during puberty. What happens precisely during puberty? There are two parts to it. There is the preparation for it, which we could call the pre-teen years, and then there is the time when the formation of sexual characteristics is complete. This is when a girl starts to menstruate. The result of puberty is the change from an infertile being to a fertile one.

This is all ruled by the endocrine system. How well a girl undergoes this change is influenced by the environment—diet, stress, and epigenetics—much more than the genetics scientists like to claim as a determinant. Historically, these changes occurred several years later than they do now. The fact that girls are menstruating younger and younger is the root of many health issues.[2]

The neuroendocrine system comprises the hypothalamus, pituitary, thyroid, and adrenal glands. Pubertal development can be thrown off its regular physiological track by any hormone not receiving proper signaling to do its job in talking to other hormones. There is a continual crosstalk between the neuroendocrine system and all tissues in the body.[3] During puberty, all hormone levels change, not only the ones you associate with being fertile. In fact, thyroid hormone is the great conductor of this orchestra of many different hormones.[4] Thyroid hormone decides when and how all the other glands secrete their hormones.[5]

The endocrine system directs the physical changes in appearance and organs. On the outside, there is pubic hair growth, breast formation, a widening of the hips, the labia minora lengthening, and a widening of the vulva. The uterus increases in dimension on the inside, and endometrial tissue, which lines the uterus, gets thicker. The ovaries also increase in size and release eggs that move through the fallopian tubes and into the uterus. Both adrenal and thyroid hormones trigger the secretion of gonadotropins that, in turn, trigger the increased secretion of sex steroids that lead to the maturation of the girl into a fertile being.[6]

This doesn't happen all at once. There is usually a growth spurt to signal the beginning of puberty. Breast tissue, the same for both boys and girls before these changes, starts to develop and eventually reaches full size for 4 to 5 years. Pubic hair is sparse at first and becomes thicker and coarser towards the end of puberty. The physical formations take several years and culminate with a girl getting her period.

Scientists have tried to create a scale and name stages of puberty in both girls and boys. In 1969, James Tanner's scale became used to indicate the timing of pubertal development from start to finish.[7] His scale has five Stages: starting at 8 and finishing at 15, going from pre-teen in Stage l to mature female in Stage lV . It describes the formation of sexual characteristics associated with puberty, such as pubic hair growth, breast development, and vulval tissue development. Its illustrations and photos have become the gold standard for measuring pubertal development.

There are two problems with the continued use of the Tanner scale. James Tanner, a British pediatrician, and R.H. Whitehouse first described the Tanner scale in 1955. Tanner, Whitehouse, and their assistant, W.A. Marshall, measured and photographed white female and male children living in an orphanage in London, England, from 1949 to 1971. At that time, only 1 % of girls were starting Stage ll at 8.

Recent global studies demonstrate that more girls are going through puberty at much younger ages. A study from the 1990s indicated that 48% of girls were at Stage ll at age 8.[8] This makes the Tanner scale obsolete.

The other problem is that these children did not have the right to refuse to be measured. It was also stressful for them. The children had to remain naked and still while pictures were being taken for quite some time. This was in the 1950s, so there were no digital cameras to speed this up. Tanner has consistently defended his studies as a means to differentiate children who were too young to be considered adults for work or even sexual slavery. He maintained that his study demonstrated that malnutrition and stress in these institutions could prevent proper development and advocated for more nutritional support for low-income families.

The Tanner Stages focused more on the physical changes during puberty, such as breast formation and pubic hair growth. They are still the foundation of the medical Sexual Maturity Rating (SMR).

Adrenarche, pubarche, thelarche, and menarche are also used to describe pubertal stages.[9]

The field of adolescent gynecology discusses puberty as having two distinct processes, which are first adrenarche, when adrenally secreted hormones that peaked at 6 months of age in babies and then plummeted, are reactivated and begin start secretion again, and gonadarche, which activates the hypothalamus and pituitary glands to produce gonadotropins.

Pubarche is the appearance of pubic hair and is considered a manifestation of adrenarche. Thelarche is the development of breast tissue. Since scientists began using Tanner Stages, clinicians have considered the beginning of breast development as the beginning of puberty in girls and have associated this stage with gonadarche. Menarche culminates with a girl's first menses.

Adrenarche occurs before the pre-teen years in girls, usually between 6-8, and is considered an endocrine preparation for puberty. During adrenarche, the adrenal cortex matures and produces dehydroepiandrosterone and dehydroepiandrosterone sulfate (DHEA and DHEAS). As the name suggests, the hormones that trigger pubertal development are androgen hormones associated with male development. This stage occurs in males and females at different times (boys go through this stage a couple of years later than girls). We now know that girls are only 5% different genetically from boys. Sex chromosomes make up only 5% of human genes.[10] There is very little biological difference between males and females. Males and females synthesize both these hormones in adrenal glands their entire lives. The degree of this synthesis pivots a fetus to form female or male sexual characteristics during the second month of fetal development.

In the last 20 years, several papers have demonstrated a pubertal stage called thyroidarche.[11] During this stage of pre-pubertal development, the thyroid gland becomes bigger and produces higher levels of T3 and T4. The conversion from the inactive thyroxine (T4) to the active triiodothyronine (T3) conversion also peaks. The pulsatile secretion of TSH in the pituitary gland increases in volume and occurs more often. Thyroid hormone production increases more in pre-teen girls than it does in boys. This is made clear by studies demonstrating that more girls than boys living in iodine-deficient areas develop goiter. This happens between 8 and 10. At 12 to 14, the hypothalamus is triggered by both thyroid and DHEA to secrete GnRH (gonadotropin-releasing hormone. GnRH signals the pituitary to increase the secretion of follicle-stimulating hormone (FSH) and luteinizing hormone (LH) which begins the gonadarche stage.

The rise in FHS stimulates an increase in estrone and estradiol, as well as the maturation of the follicles in the ovaries that produce eggs. LH regulates the synthesis of progesterone, which is necessary for the maturation of the uterine endometrium for the implantation of a fertilized egg.

Several papers have pointed out that clinical dependence on Tanner staging and Sexual Maturity Rating (SMR) may lead to misdiagnoses of precocious puberty or delayed puberty and parental and teen concern that they are not passing through these stages properly. The United States National Library of Medicine (NIH) states that Tanner staging "is an objective classification system that providers use to document and track the development and sequence of secondary sex characteristics of children during puberty."[12] The problem is that Western medicine depends on these stages from research garnered from studying white children in the West at a time when people ate quite differently than they do now. These children did not avoid eating animal products or animal fat as many pubertal girls have since the 1980s. Nor did Tanner's research consider different diets that include large amounts of plant sterols, such as millet and sweet potato, which raise estrogen, testosterone, and progesterone levels just as much as birth control medications. Tanner's research followed

260 girls, but only 48 were followed for ten years, from pre-teen years to the completion of puberty.

Some girls have pubarche before thelarche, and some the other way around. In one study, non-Hispanic white girls had breast development before pubic hair, while non-Hispanic black girls developed breasts before pubic hair. Another research paper studied Danish teenage girls and found that girls who first had thelarche before pubarche had lower birth weights and were born prematurely.[13]

There isn't a right way for a girl to develop during puberty. The development can be different for every girl and depends on various factors. Some girls may get pubic hair before their breasts mature. Some girls' vulvas may grow differently than others. Tanner and his assistant Marshall spent years photographing the physical development of these few white English girls' breasts, vulval, and pubic hair growth development. His stages were incorporated into what is used today as in pediatric and gynecological Sexual Maturity Rating (SMR). I don't find it objective, based on so few subjects. I can imagine any girl looking at these photos and illustrations and wondering why she doesn't match the exact development dictated by the scale.

Gynecologists and pediatricians use these images to measure whether a girl is developing correctly. They may conclude erroneously that a girl is developing too slowly or too quickly and prescribe hormones. At the very least, this conclusion can make a girl self-conscious and think there is something wrong with her development, even though there may be nothing wrong. Some teenage girls will seek labiaplasty to have their vulval tissue look more like the images they see on the Tanner scale. This can lead to mutilation by plastic surgeons who are not educated adequately in female clitoral anatomy.

Female anatomy has always been deemed a low priority by medicine. The image of the female clitoris was erased from medical textbooks in the 20th century. There has only been an anatomically correct image of the clitoris since 1981. In 2005, Australian urologist Helen

O'Connell was so infuriated at conducting surgery without any anatomical information comparable to what is found in textbooks on the penis, she developed a 3D rendering of the clitoris.[14]

Jessica Ann Pin's work has demonstrated that the anatomy of clitoral nerves is missing from obstetrical-gynecological textbooks.[15] She is an influential activist who is working to have textbooks revised to include anatomically correct drawings so surgeons will not cut through nerves and cause women to lose the ability to orgasm, something that happened to her during a labiaplasty surgery. She also educates young women that labial tissue is different for all women, and labiaplasty, the world's fast-growing aesthetic surgery being performed by surgeons ignorant of female anatomy, is seldom even necessary. There is no right way for vulval tissue to look.

Many parts of this normal physiological development can be thrown off track. The neuroendocrine system depends on proper signaling.[16] Genetic aberrations are rare. A genetic disorder due to an extra X chromosome in girls can cause Turner syndrome, the symptoms of which are short height, heart problems, and the absence of ovarian development. Turner syndrome is rare, affecting 1 in 2000 girls.[17]

Some problems may be caused by environmental xenoestrogens, medications with steroid hormones, and even foods with phytosterols, such as sweet potato and soy. Most physicians and parents are concerned about either precocious or delayed puberty. Often, medications are prescribed to hasten or prevent pubertal maturation, which causes further endocrine imbalances and affects the endocrine health for the rest of a woman's life. There are also many symptoms of dysregulated pubertal development, such as PCOS and endometriosis, that are on the rise and occurring in younger girls.

The endocrine changes that come with puberty are straightforward. Humans evolved to go through these changes without any problems. The perils of puberty are something new that came into the social and medical discourse less than two hundred years ago, and these perils are only associated with girls. This fact in itself should make a girl wonder why she is being prescribed antidepressants and hormones when boys are not. Despite Joe Jackson's song, "It's Different for Girls," it isn't really, not physically, anyway. Society and culture have made it different for girls. I wish I had some of the songs to listen to that girls have access to today. Songs by women were mainly about love. Songs by men were more political.

Just a few Ska bands wrote about things besides love when I was an adolescent. I've told my daughters many times that I wish women's hip-hop had been playing on the radio when I was a teenager. The biases in medicine also exist in the music industry. Of course, they do since men have historically dominated all industries. A female songwriter bemoans stereotypes in the industry "of the romantic, vulnerable, adorable girl on the one side, and the sexy tiger on the other."[18] This sounds precisely like the dichotomy created during the mid-19th century I described in the previous chapter. She writes, "We rarely hear women songwriters singing about politics or our society. Women artists are often expected to write and sing about one theme: love, either in its romantic and mushy declination or its explicitly sexual meaning."[19] As a recent *New York Times* article titled "The Future of Rap Is Female," young female rap artists have turned sexual objectification "on its head."[20] It's refreshing and empowering. It's the only music I listen to at 61.

FOUR

THE CAUSES OF HEALTH ISSUES DURING PUBERTY

BARRING TUMORS OR PATHOLOGY, HEALTH issues during puberty are caused by a combination of nutritional deficiency and endocrine imbalance. Any deficiency in essential nutrients will also cause an endocrine imbalance. The development of sexual characteristics that define puberty will not happen without issue if any element required for a smooth physiological transition from childhood to adulthood is missing. The word hormone comes from the Greek word *hormōn*, which means to set in motion. The endocrine system is a network of glands that regulate metabolism, energy, growth, development, and the immune and stress response. The entire system uses hormones for organs, cells, and tissues to communicate with glands and vice versa. I will outline three essential components that are causing the complicated steps of the journey of a female child to a female adolescent to go wrong. I will discuss how crucial dietary is for this transition to be smooth. If there isn't an adequate level of iodine, an essential nutrient long-maligned, demonized, and ignored by medicine, puberty will be fraught with the health issues I discussed in the previous chapter, for which medicines with terrible side effects are prescribed. Finally, thyroid gland secretion and adrenal gland secretion, for which dietary fat and iodine are fundamental to proper function, are the foundation for healthy pubertal development.

Thyroid Function and Diet

The first stage of puberty is the thyroidarche. This means the thyroid begins to produce more of its hormones to initiate the growth and development of sexual characteristics. The active thyroid hormone is T3, which, in this instance, functions as a growth hormone to initiate the formation of breasts, the growth of pubic hair, and the enlargement of the reproductive organs—the ovaries and the uterus. Thyroid hormone stimulates the adrenal cortex to increase in size and to increase the secretion of androgen hormones needed for the subsequent stage in puberty, that of adrenarche. Thyroid hormones also signal the hypothalamic-pituitary-ovarian (HPO) axis, which regulates ovarian production of estrogen and progesterone.[1]

What does the thyroid need to be able to produce hormones? Besides iodine, which provides the raw material from which thyroid hormones are constructed (which I will discuss further), it needs specific vitamins, amino acids, and minerals. Without iron, selenium, and zinc, thyroid hormone biosynthesis, metabolism, and action will be limited. Vitamin B12 and B2 are essential for thyroid function. Trace minerals such as zinc, copper, chromium, calcium, and selenium must be sufficient, but excess trace minerals will damage thyroid function.[2] Selenium is crucial for the conversion of T4 to the active T3. But too much will lower T3 levels in circulation.[3] Zinc is also essential for the conversion of T4 to T3. Too much calcium lowers thyroid hormone levels.[4] A copper deficiency causes less tyrosine to be synthesized. Tyrosine is an amino acid precursor to iodine-based thyroid hormones—T4, T3, T2, and T1. You can see it's all about balancing these nutrients. Taking them in less bioavailable forms from supplements can put a wrench in the works.

Tyrosine is an amino acid derived from phenylalanine, another amino acid. Other thyroid-important amino acids are carnitine, valine, leucine, arginine, asparagine, and serine. All are needed for proper thyroid function. Low carnitine is associated with higher thyroid antibodies. Serine modulates the secretion of TSH in the brain. Calcitonin, another hormone produced in the thyroid that regulates calcium levels is made out of 32 different amino acids.[5] Since Vitamin D is an immune system modulator, a deficiency in it is associated with higher thyroid antibodies.[6] However, high levels of Vitamin A correlate with lower TSH expression. Iron is essential because it converts T4 into T3 using thyroid peroxidase. For this reason, a diet has to provide the most bioavailable sources of these nutrients. It must not contain foods that contain anti-nutrients, preventing the metabolism of the nutrients listed above.

Many plants contain anti-nutrients that prevent the absorption of minerals and vitamins and goitrogens that prevent the absorption of iodine. The family of Brassica vegetables, which includes cabbage, broccoli, bok choy, oat, soy, millet, cassava, and yams, contain chemicals that have been isolated to prevent the thyroid from taking in iodine, commonly known today as the anti-thyroid medication Methimazole.[7] This occurred when a farmer noticed that his rabbits who ate cabbage leaves developed goiter.[8] Lemon balm (Melissa officinalis) and the herb rosemary lower thyroid hormone levels.

Thyroid hormones are made out of the amino acid tyrosine and iodine molecules. Without iodine, the endocrine system cannot proceed appropriately during puberty, as puberty starts with adequate thyroid function signaling. Iodine deficiency is a global emergency.

Not only are congenital learning disabilities associated with iodine deficiency, but more girls than boys are deficient in iodine. This has been known since David Marine's research in Akron, Ohio, an area part of the US upper Midwest goiter belt in the 1920s. He studied 2000 girls and saw that 200 mg of sodium iodide intake for 5th to 8th-grade girls and 400 mg for older girls prevented goiter.[9]

Iodized salt contains a small amount of iodine in the form of sodium iodide, but this quickly evaporates. Iodized salt, while preventing goiter, does not provide enough iodine to prevent low thyroid function, which leads to inadequate hormone signaling and a cascade of hormone imbalances that will lead to the health issues during puberty I prescribed previously. The absence of goiter does not mean adequate iodine for thyroid function. Marine's 9 mg of iodine in the form of sodium iodide only prevented goiter. It did not improve grades or reduce school absences due to illness.[10]

The thyroid prefers potassium iodide to elemental iodine. Still, the tissues girls build during puberty—a growing uterus, growing ovaries, growing breasts, growing labia minora, and pubic hair, need elemental iodine.[11] Iodized salt does not provide elemental iodine.[12] Whereas a hundred years ago, most iodine deficiencies were associated with mountainous goiter belt regions, in countries and states such as Switzerland, parts of Italy, Michigan, and Tennessee mountain areas, physicians since Caleb Parry in 1808 noted that stress was commonly associated with goiter.[13]

Today, since the addition of halides such as fluoride to many municipal water supplies, and bromide to foods, plastics, and household items, and the inevitability of exposure to forever chemicals such as phthalates and BPAs in water, chemicals, and cosmetics, which all interfere with the absorption of iodine, it is nearly impossible for anyone on planet earth to be sufficient in iodine.[14] Many medications and supplements generally interfere with iodine absorption and thyroid function.[15] Quercetin is an excellent example of this. This popular supplement inhibits thyroid gland tissue's thyroid cell growth and iodine uptake.[16] Of the medications commonly prescribed to children and teenagers, cortisone and cortisone inhalers, dopamine agonists suppress TSH and lower the conversion of T4 to T3.[17] Retinoids, prescribed for acne, also suppress TSH.[18] Tricyclic antidepressants, such as Prozac, are prescribed to treat depression.[19] Lithium is commonly prescribed to treat children and teenagers with depression and bipolar disorder.[20] These drugs lower iodine absorption and decrease the TSH response to Thyroid-regulating hormone (TRH). Metformin, commonly prescribed for weight control and diabetes, suppresses TSH. Immunosuppressants increase cause the production of thyroid antibodies.[21] Since a study demonstrated that thyroid hormone metabolism and human chorionic gonadotropin secretion increased in healthy pregnant women HCG injections became part of weight loss programs.[22]

After these studies emerged, British physician Albert T. Simeons promoted injections of HCG and a 500-calorie diet to burn body fat, like the horrible little book I found in the bookstore when I was 15. Both the HCG injections and severe calorie restriction would lower thyroid hormone levels so that tissues would not be able to get what they need. Dr. Richard Lipman's website promotes his "modified 800 calorie HCG-Like Diet for teens from 13-17." He sells kits on his website containing syringes and bottles of human chorionic gonadotropin.[23]

At the same time as Evelyn Mann's research demonstrating that low iodine levels in pregnant women caused learning disorders in their babies,[24] Wolff-Chaikoff's erroneous conclusion that iodine caused hypothyroidism in rodents in 1948 caused the subsequent demonization of iodine.[25] Since the Wolff-Chaikoff debacle, all nations have reduced the required daily intake of iodine to 150 mcg in adults and only 120 mcg in preteens and adolescents. Thyroid gland or goiter enlargement prevalence due to iodine deficiency in adolescent females remains, even in iodine-sufficient regions, as a Belgian researcher stated, "a puzzling problem."[26] The real problem is that researchers are looking at goiter as the sole symptom of iodine deficiency. What is clear is that thyroid hormones rise significantly during adolescence and more so in girls than boys.[27] Iodine is necessary to manufacture those thyroid hormones. At about 9 years of age, iodine levels plummet by 25%.[28] This means a preteen female needs a minimum of a 25% increase in iodine intake at the beginning of puberty.

Menstruation requires more iodine.[29] A 15% increase is necessary during menstruation. The ovaries, which grow during puberty next to the thyroid and breast tissue, need large amounts of iodine. Female adolescents need more iodine than males due to the needs of the tissues associated with reproduction. Any deficiency will cause these tissues to try to trap more iodine and cause a hyperplastic response, exactly like goiter in the thyroid, in the form of fibroids and cysts. [30]

Low-Fat and Hypocaloric Diets

Adolescence is when many females start to diet. Breasts get bigger, and hips widen. Unrealistic conceptions about beauty—I say this because I, too, felt the pressure to be thin and willowy during adolescence, and I too took to semi-starvation to achieve this goal—will make girls avoid the foods our culture tells us are fattening. Those foods, meat, and fat, are precisely what the growing pubertal female needs. Women have been convinced that because carbohydrates have fewer calories than meat and fat, avoiding them will help them achieve the slender body associated with beauty. From the 1950s to the 1970s, the sugar lobby in the United States marketed it as a healthy nutrient that would curb hunger and boost energy. Fat and meat have been demonized because they contain cholesterol, which Ancel Key's sham study claimed to demonstrate in 1958 caused heart disease.[31] The metabolic changes required to build the sexual characteristics of puberty need both of these nutrients in abundance.

The first stage of puberty is the thyroidarche. Thyroid hormone production needs not only fat-soluble vitamins, such as vitamin D (found only in cholesterol), the minerals and amino acids discussed above, but adequate caloric intake or T4, the inactive thyroid hormone, will not be converted into T3, but reverse T3. This is because thyroid hormone regulates metabolism and growth. No tissues, cells, enzymes, or hormones can be fabricated with inadequate nutrition. Functional physiology decreases. The factory has to shut down, and budget cuts to a business force it to manufacture less due to the lack of raw materials. It is important to note that this is a question of calories and nutrition. Foods devoid of nutrition but full of calories will not turn on the conveyor belt. Much is written about the importance of carbohydrates for thyroid function, but this is not true. Inadequate nutrition lowers thyroid hormone levels. A diet higher in fat calories demonstrated increased thyroid function when compared to a diet with the same calories derived from carbohydrates.[32]

The androgen hormones needed to stimulate the adrenarche stage of puberty require the production of steroid hormones. This is when dehydroepiandrosterone sulfate (DHEAS) and cortisol secretion increase in the adrenal cortex due to increased ACTH from the pituitary. The DHEA and DHEAS are precursor hormones. Peripheral conversion in all tissues is what brings about the physiological changes of adrenarche, such as in hair follicles (pubic and axillary hair growth), genital skin (the enlargement of labia minora tissue, and a moderate increase in body odor, and sebaceous gland production. After a surge in adrenal hormone production at birth, these hormone levels plummet until adrenarche, where steroidogenesis ramps up.

Steroidogenesis is the process through which cholesterol (only derived from dietary animal fat and liver synthesis) is converted to steroid hormones.[33] This development includes the beginning of pubic hair growth called pubarche in the Tanner stages. DHEAS and other androgen hormones are also associated with brain neuroplasticity, a growth spurt, and sebaceous and apocrine gland development in the skin. An imbalance of adrenal hormone production can lead to acne and pimples associated with adolescence. An imbalance at this time will also cause precocious puberty, which occurs 5 to 9 times more in girls than boys.[34] Premature adrenarche is associated with hirsutism, acne, increased body odor, oily hair, and skin.

Higher ACTH secretion and the increased volume of the adrenal glands after thyroidarche also cause cortisol levels to increase. Diseases such as Addison's cause low cortisol levels due to adrenal tumors preventing cortisol production, demonstrating the absence of adrenarche and the development of puberty, and Cushing's Syndrome, which causes high cortisol levels and premature adrenarche and pubarche due to androgen hormone synthesis, represent the extremes.

However, a child can manifest both illnesses if cortisol levels are too low or too high, even without adrenal tissue disorders. The adrenal glands and gonads are the primary sources of steroid hormones.[35] If steroid hormone production is essential to steroidogenesis, a low-fat diet will cause an imbalance. The liver produces cholesterol, but the physiological need for cholesterol is so great that dietary cholesterol is crucial for healthy steroidogenesis.

One of the causes of an imbalance is a diet low in fat but also a carbohydrate diet. High insulin levels raise cortisol levels but also disrupt steroidogenesis.[36] A diet high in carbohydrates and low in fat will increase insulin and cortisol levels. The enzyme aromatase is found in many tissues, such as blood, adipose, and bone tissue, and is crucial to converting one steroid hormone into another along the steroid hormone cascade. High cortisol, high insulin levels, and xenoestrogens can disrupt this conversion. Since stress also raises cortisol, any trauma, inflammation, overexercise, and use of stimulants will also affect the endocrine system's ability to regulate hormone production and signaling.[37] The stress and immune response are made out of cholesterol.[38]

Dieting is in itself a stress. Cortisol levels will rise with malnourishment, just as they will with overexercise. I remember the little book I had that listed different foods and the calories they contained. One time, I ate two cookies and ran up and down the stairs of my mother's townhouse until enough time had passed for me to have supposedly burnt the amount of calories the two cookies contained. Girls who overtrain on sports teams lose their cycle. Those girls are carb-loading before events, as my older daughter did with her teammates on her crew team, but they are not eating animal fat. Potato chips and Oreo cookies are unsaturated when used to contain lard. However, since lard has cholesterol, food companies increased the sugar content of packaged foods and substituted the lard for unsaturated fatty acids or trans fats made of vegetable oil. Trans fats are highly inflammatory, and while the medical establishment has finally reached the same conclusion, the population has been told to avoid these foods and eat more polyunsaturated fats that contain nut oils and seed oils, which are unfortunately just as inflammatory as the unsaturated fats. Hormones cannot be made out of these substances.

The recommendations to avoid meat and animal fat come from the same misguided ideas from the Victorian Era that created the weak and depressed female girl. Today's US dietary guidelines originated from people who were Seventh-Day Adventists. This anti-meat agenda cannot be traced back to promoting improved health, preventing chronic disease, or sustaining life on Earth. There are potent lobbies behind the anti-meat campaign by Ellen G. White, who established the church based on her visions. Members of this church founded processed food companies that today have become huge global conglomerates that fund and push their religious ideology of a plant-based diet on the rest of us through dietary guidelines, shoddy research, and publicity campaigns.[39]

They have the world's most extensive nonprofit healthcare system as part of their evangelical efforts. This includes hospitals, sanitariums, nursing homes, retirement homes, orphanages, and universities. The Adventist Health International is based in Loma Linda, California. John Harvey Kellogg, who developed the breakfast cereal, medicalized and secularized the Seventh-Day Adventist church as a means in and of itself.[40] Not only does the SDA church have universities that focus on nutrition in wellness in the US, but it has founded them all over the world. All the meat substitute foods in health food stores are derived from soybeans in the United States and started as Kellogg products. They have received over $24 million in funding from the National Institutes of Health since 2002. The result has been over 110 peer-reviewed publications. Over the last 50 years, influential medical journals such as *JAMA*, *The New England Journal of Medicine*, and the *Archives of Internal Medicine* have published on subjects promoting the benefits of a vegetarian diet, from eating nuts to the diet and prostate cancer, diet and type 2 diabetes, and diet and cancer, heart disease and mortality.[41]

The Adventist involvement and influence on public dietary advice started with Lenna Francis Cooper, a protégé of Dr. John Harvey Kellogg, who founded the American Dietetic Association (ADA) in 1917. Lenna Cooper was a leading proponent of health care through diet and a highly influential Adventist dietitian, with more than 500 dietitians graduating from Battle Creek Sanitarium under her tutelage.[42] She was the first US Army dietitian and served on the staff of the US Surgeon General created the dietetics department at the National Institutes of Health.[43]

She was the senior author of *Nutrition in Health and Disease*, a textbook used for 30 years in diet and nursing programs worldwide.

When Ancel Keys published his seven countries study, he claimed that saturated fat, found in animal fat, caused heart disease. At the same time, Doctor Yudkin, a British nutritionist and former Chair of Nutrition at Queen Elizabeth College in London, insisted that sugar, not cholesterol, was the cause of heart disease.[44] His book,

Pure, White, and Deadly, was the first book written by a scientist since William Banting's small book, *Letter On Corpulence*, published in 1863, to warn about the adverse health effects of the public's increased sugar consumption following fat's vilification. He suffered a barrage of criticism then, particularly from the sugar industry and processed food manufacturers. The massive growth of the processed food industry is linked to John Harvey Kellogg's feat of merchandising meat substitutes that all began as a way of preventing people from having carnal desires. Ancel Keys, the American physiologist, had his cholesterol hypothesis debunked when it was revealed that he falsified his research and argued in favor of restricting dietary fat, not sugar.[45] It incited the medical establishment to ridicule Yudkin's work.[46]

The 1977 US McGovern Report and subsequent dietary Goals for the United States were heavily influenced by the Sugar Research Foundation and Seventh-day Adventist ideology. We know this because Nathan Pritikin, creator of the Pritikin Diet, a low-fat, high-fiber diet, was a close friend of Senator George McGovern and an adjunct professor at the Adventist Loma Linda University.[47] He acknowledged reading Ellen G White's writings in the 1940s and became a vocal advocate of low-fat, 'plant-based' diets.[48]

Adventist Hans Diehl, founder of CHIP, was the Director of Education and Research at the Pritikin Longevity Centre from 1976.[49] He founded The Complete Health Improvement Program (CHIP) as a premier lifestyle intervention targeting chronic disease with a primarily plant-based, whole-food diet and regular exercise. Senator McGovern's aide, Nick Mottern, is said to have been an Adventist and a vegetarian when he wrote the Dietary Goals for the United States in 1977. Seventh-day Adventists would be in control of the dietary guidelines for the United States from then.

The 'fear of fat' worked its way into the medical curriculum in the 80s, teaching generations of medical professionals to "fear cholesterol," something so utterly vital to life that our bodies make it.

The rest of the world followed suit—adopting the same plant-based, anti-meat rhetoric as a preventative and curative way of eating. Since the implementation of these anti-meat, pro-grain guidelines, the rate of diabetes has skyrocketed in the US and globally.[50, 51] The Seventh-day Adventists created Lifestyle Medicine, which soon teamed up with Coca-Cola and other global conglomerates to ensure people continue to consume more processed food devoid of essential nutrients.[52]

By the 21st century, neither the sinfulness of masturbation, the health warnings that meat causes cancer, nor the worry that cattle are diseased made the impact on non-believers the church was campaigning for. The Seventh-day Adventist Church refocused its anti-meat campaign to align with "Climate Change." By blending religion, science, philosophy, and politics, the Seventh-day Adventist Church has been able to establish a scientific rationale for vegetarianism and align itself with powerful lobby groups—vegans and the food industry.[53] Now, nutrition science implicates meat eating as not just harming people but also harming the planet.

A research paper into how females and males perceive climate change differently concluded that males focus more on science and business arguments and that women are more concerned with policies related to ethics and justice. The paper states that men "showed gender matching tendencies" because they focused on the more historically "masculine" discourse of science and business since men are more associated with science and technology.[54] This is because women have been traditionally denied entry into fields of science and technology, not because it doesn't interest them. Women weren't allowed to study anything until the 20th century. Women weren't initially allowed to practice even if they graduated from medical or law school. Hypatia, one of the only recorded female mathematicians, was also an astronomer and philosopher who taught at an influential school of philosophy in Alexandria. She was murdered by, according to her contemporary, the Greek Christian historian Socrates of Constantinople, by a Christian mob in 415.[55]

The dichotomy between what is male and what is female was created by society in the late 18th century. This dichotomy deepened during the 19th century. There is only a 5% genetic difference between males and females.[56] This is not enough to make women more interested in ethics and justice and men more interested in science and business. It is a cultural creation that has been and continues to be upheld by medicine and commerce. What is essential is that females build more sexual characteristics than men, which requires more tissue development, meaning females need more iodine and dietary fat than men.

Women avoid eating fat. Men don't. Even though their doctors tell them to avoid meat and fat, men keep eating it. There are countless studies in the current climate when we are told to avoid eating meat initially for our health. The Seventh Day Adventists have a lot to do with this. and over the last few years, for the planet. But we cannot blame it entirely on them. High rates of diabetes mean one sells a lot of insulin. High rates of depression mean many antidepressants are sold. Claiming endocrine issues are to blame for health issues in women rakes in the money.[57]

FIVE

MEDICINES FOR PUBERTY

ARE THE HEALTH ISSUES THAT girls have during puberty and adolescence treated differently today than they were in the 19th century? You would think that with all the scientific advances we have seen in medicine, treating a hormonal imbalance caused by nutritional deficiencies, stress, and toxins would not be treated with dangerous chemicals or surgery. Unfortunately, this is not the case in the treatment of puberty issues and behavioral and mental health issues of adolescence, nor is it the case of the same form of treatment for the same symptoms associated with menopause, as I discuss in my first book, *Good Fat is Good for Women: Menopause*.[1]

We can compare the language used by physicians of the mid-to-end 19th century with the language of scientists today. At the end of the 19th century, a massive amount of medical articles were published that discussed the diseases and disorders of women that were seen as connected to the reproductive process. Girls were seen as invalids because they had a menstrual cycle, which was seen as making them prone to disease. As this disease process was primarily seen in middle and upper-class women, it is clear that this is a cultural construction and not a biological one. In her paper "Exercise, Physical Capability, and the Eternally Wounded Woman in Late Nineteenth Century North America," Patricia Vertinsky shows how these arguments "increasingly defined medical views of women's health and the productive boundaries of their lives."[2]

American physician Edward Clarke published a book against educating girls called *Sex in Education or A Fair Chance for the Girls in 1873*, arguing that "'from school or college excellent scholars, but with underdeveloped ovaries."[3] In psychiatrist Henry Maudsley's article in 1874 called "Sex in Mind and in Education," published in the *Fortnightly Review*, wrote that "They cannot choose but to be women: cannot rebel successfully against the tyranny of their organization, the complete development and function whereof must take place after its kind. . .That the development of puberty does draw heavily upon the vital resources of the female constitution, needs not to be pointed out to those who know the nature of the important physiological changes which then take place. In persons of delicate constitution who have inherited a tendency to disease, and who have little vitality to spare, the disease is apt to break out at that time; the new drain established having deprived the constitution of the vital energy necessary to withstand the enemy that was lurking in it."[4]

This is an example of the language used today in a 2013 paper entitled "Menarche, Puberty and Psychiatric Disorders," published in the medical journal *Gynecological Endocrinology*: "Women are more risky about psychiatric complaints than men particularly during almost all reproductive cycles and also during adolescence. Depression is the best representative example which is more common in woman than in men and it particularly occurs at times of hormonal fluctuations. A hormonal triad of premenstrual depression, postnatal depression and climacteric depression is recently defined which is best referred to as 'reproductive depression."[5]

That women are susceptible to mental health issues due to their gender is an idea that was created in the 19th century, yet few physicians examine or question this bias. Criminal Justice historian Ellen Dwyer wrote about "the ease with which 19th century lunatic asylums could be used to control the behavior of deviant members of society, particularly females. Although families initiated the institutionalization process in most cases, the writings of medical doctors on madness and its treatment clearly justified such actions. Few contemporary psychologists look critically at the value systems that underline their work or at the intellectual roots that have fed it.[6]

Some forms of clitoral surgery continued to be performed until the mid-1990s. Today, due to the continued attempt of young women to conform to an idea of "correct" femininity that evolved due to social upheaval in the 19th century, labiaplasty is the fastest-growing aesthetic surgery worldwide.[7] Teens are concerned with the appropriate appearance of their genitalia. Women are concerned with both the appearance and sexual enhancement that clitoral surgeries have touted since the mid-19th century. Plastic surgeons and gynecologists today use the same arguments that surgeons and gynecologists used then. Women who have these surgeries experience frequent urinary tract infections, vulval dryness, and often the loss of clitoral stimulation.[8]

Concern over the rise of what some publications have called the desire for the "designer vagina"[9] in girls as young as nine has many plastic surgeons on the defensive, explaining that larger than "normal" labia minora cause pain during sex, discomfort during exercise and when donning swimsuits or tight clothing, in spite there being no research proving this.[10] A paper by plastic surgeons from 2017, which sought to address the criticism from various fields condemning the rise in the surgery, stated, "Part of our work should be focused on examining the various aesthetic and functional complaints encountered by patients who have enlarged labia minora."[11]

But women don't have enlarged labia. There is no such thing as a size that constitutes normal. It is called vaginal rejuvenation when advertised to older women. The language plastic surgeons use, such as calling the labial tissue "flaps," makes it seem like the tissue is something extra that could be easily shorn.[12] The procedure choices include the same clitoral hood reduction surgeons used in the 1900s to prevent masturbation, insanity, hysteria, and nymphomania. Thousands of women are maimed by uneducated plastic surgeons who haven't been taught clitoral anatomy in medical school to ensure they will not sever nerves essential to orgasm.[13, 14] Plastic surgery capitalizes on the age-old fear that a woman has to look like the male fantasy of a docile middle-class white female way to be attractive.

Surgeries are not promoted only for aesthetic reasons. Girls and women are told that surgical removal of the clitoral hood will enhance their sexual pleasure. Yet women with normal clitorises do not have any issues having an orgasm. The issue that has been invented is that women, according to the surgeons who started performing the surgeries in the mid-19th century, is that women will more easily have an orgasm the "correct" way with vaginal penetration.[15] There is plenty of research that proves most women do not orgasm with vaginal penetration.[16] This has been seen as a drawback because women orgasming without penetration would mean men were not necessary for the sexual act. The female clitoris has always been known as the main organ for women's sexual pleasure, but physicians have always seen it as a failed penis.[17] It works much like a penis. It swells during stimulation and needs to be stimulated, but physicians, unaware of the anatomy of this female genital organ, thought it relatively puny, compared to the male penis.

The idea of women getting sexual pleasure without vaginal penetration was disturbing to the male physicians in the mid-19th century.[18]

Separating female sexuality from childbearing was seen as sinful. Hence, it was reasoned that removing the clitoral hood to liberate the clitoris would increase a female's sensitivity to the male organ and thus ensure her orgasm during intercourse with her husband. This did not work. Females who had had their clitoris surgically altered often would not be able to have any pleasure at all, as the nerves were often severed during surgery. Medical historian Sara B. Rodriguez wrote that "Over the course of 150 years, physicians performed—and some women, their spouses, and parents of girls sought out—clitoral surgeries to maintain or conform to the sexual behavior deemed culturally appropriate for women."[19]

Dangerous surgeries aside, there are many medications prescribed to girls and young women that seek to address the health issues associated with puberty and adolescence that continue the medical trend that started in the 19th century. The crucial point is that these are not prescribed to boys going through puberty at the rate at which they are prescribed to girls. Birth control has never been prescribed to boys. The only birth control that exists for boys is the condom. There is one new hormonal drug being investigated called Dimethandrolone undecanoate (DMAU), that would need to be taken daily. However, the known side effects (long-term studies have not been done) are similar to what they are for the female version—headaches, weight gain, erectile dysfunction, and loss of libido—so it is not yet on the market.[20] Then why has it been on the market for women since the isolation of steroid hormones in the 1930s? Men have traditionally refused to take birth control. A 2016 study was halted due to men reporting effects on their mood.[21] Another medication was rejected because the testicles of the men taking part in the study shrunk. No birth control tested on women was ever rejected due to side effects of mood swings to cancer.

Menstruation

Puberty culminates with menstruation. The endocrine system has been busy in the background since the preteen years, beginning with the thyroidarche, then the adrenarche, and finishing with gonadarche. Menstruation signifies that follicle-stimulating hormones have signaled an increase in estrone and estradiol and the growth of the follicles in the ovaries that will produce eggs. An egg will pass into the fallopian tubes, waiting for sperm to be fertilized. Luteinizing hormone begins regulating the synthesis of progesterone, which is necessary for the maturation of the uterine endometrium for the implantation of a fertilized egg.

The body is now ready for the menstrual cycle, which takes an average of 28 days. The cycle begins with menses when the uterus sheds the tissue that thickens in preparation for a fertilized egg. The uterine tissue moves out of the uterus, through the cervix, and into the vaginal canal in the form of blood to pass out of the body. This phase usually lasts from three to five days.

The follicular phase follows the menses or what we now mostly call the period. This phase lasts from about day 6 to day 14. The estrogen level then rises to renew the thickening of the uterine tissue. Follicle-stimulating hormone stimulates the ovaries to produce eggs. Finally, the Luteal phase, from day 15-28, causes the egg to leave the ovary and travel to the fallopian tubes to the uterus in case there is sperm to fertilize it. Progesterone rises to prepare the endometrium, the tissue that lines the uterus, for possible pregnancy. Pregnancy occurs if sperm fertilizes the eggs. If this does not occur, both estrogen and progesterone levels fall, and the uterus sheds again, resulting in menstrual blood and the beginning of a new cycle.

A more straightforward explanation would be that menstruation is the breakdown of uterine tissue when estrogen and progesterone are both low. Then follows a regeneration phase, where first estrogen rises at about day 10 and then progesterone at about day 14. There is then a secretion phase from day 14 to day 28 that causes endometrial tissue to thicken. Finally, the estrogen and progesterone both fall again to cause menstruation.

Although FSH, LH, progesterone, and estrogen are crucial for menstruation, no hormone functions in isolation. There is constant crosstalk between hormones, which turns signaling on or off. The body does not want anything to go wrong. Malnutrition is one example of what could cause the negative feedback response that is involved in all physiological processes to prevent menstruation or cause any issues with menstruation, or any issue for that matter. Thyroid and adrenal hormone regulation is involved in the hormonal crosstalk, ensuring everything proceeds as our biology dictates.

Menstruation is not supposed to cause any symptoms. A female is supposed to look down and see that she is bleeding. There should not be a week of discomfort, mood swings, cramps, insomnia, food cravings, bloating, breast tenderness, acne, or other symptoms associated with menstruation. One of these symptoms indicates an interference or communication issue between hormones.

Precocious Puberty

At the end of the 19th century, the median age for the onset of menstruation was 15 to 16. In 1981, Marjorie Shostack documented that the earliest women in the !Kung hunter-gatherer tribes would start to menstruate at 16.[22] Today, girls as young as 8 can start menstruation. Entrepreneur parents have started special underwear for children who menstruate at such a young age. Medicine has normalized precocious menstruation despite indicating an unhealthy endocrine imbalance.

The female body evolved to menstruate several years later, yet if a girl does not menstruate at the age of 15, it is considered late, and she may very well be given hormones to trigger her cycle. The online medical reference site WebMD advises that if a girl hasn't gotten her period at 15, she should make an appointment with a doctor to determine the causes of the delay. Today, not menstruating by 15 is considered amenorrhea. A current paper stated that the absence of menstruation at age 15 was primary amenorrhea with sexual characteristics or at age 13 without the formation of sexual characteristics.[23] While medicine does agree that the cycles may be irregular for several years, this is what young women are seeing when they google at what age they should start menstruating.

Sexual characteristics are also starting to form at younger ages. According to the US Centers for Disease Control and Prevention, the average age of menstruation in the US is now 12. One hundred years ago, it was 14. Research indicates that the menarche age of menarche fell from 17 to 12 from the 1890s to the 1950s.[24] While these dramatic changes were explained as a consequence of supposedly better nutrition, the fact that in the last 20 years, the average has become even earlier is raising alarm. The first couple of years after menses begin, cycles are usually anovulatory. The possibility that a 9 and 10-year-old can become pregnant is worrisome, with some scientists raising concern that the lower age is also related to xenoestrogens found in cosmetics, everyday household items, and our water supply.[25, 26] But it also raises several health concerns.

In the mid-1990s, pediatricians were shocked to find that 17,000 American girls had started developing breasts at 10 and 9 years of age.[27] The age of puberty has been dropping by 3 months every decade from 1970 to 2013. Many doctors are stuck in the past. A paper on abnormal uterine bleeding in adolescents referenced a 2019 paper that declared that the age of menarche has remained constant at 12-13 years when both anecdotal and scientific research illustrates the opposite.[28]

While this is alarming, some doctors think the Tanner scale, which indicates the onset of puberty starts at 8 years old in girls, should be reduced to 6.[29] What could be described as the new normal was previously considered caused by either trauma or tumors in the brain triggering abnormal hormone signaling. Yet the researchers in several studies scanned the brains of pubertal girls younger than 8 and found only 1.8 % had any brain abnormalities.[30]

In the US, early puberty was initially associated with lower socio-economic status, race differences, and obesity.[31] However, since the research exploded after the shocking revelations found by pediatricians in the mid-1990s, other countries, namely Denmark, which doesn't have the same demographic, have also researched younger pubertal development.[32]

The issue with the early formation of sexual characteristics and early menstruation is that these girls are still children. They are physically becoming women when they should not yet be gendered. The 8 and 9-year-olds with breasts will be subjected to sexualization, which is hard enough for girls at 15 to deal with. Girls with early puberty have been seen to be at a higher risk of depression and anxiety than girls who reach puberty later.[33]

A mother and two daughters who started menstruating at 8 and 9 developed reusable period underwear called Girl With Big Dreams.[34] It is indeed admirable to remove the stigma of girls using products like tampons and pads during menstruation, something I remember very well from growing up. Unfortunately, many of the new reusable period pants may contain PFAS, like Goretex, which is one of the xenoestrogens that may be causing earlier menstruation.[35] Further research has shown that newer sanitary pads and tampons also contain xenoestrogens.[36]

University of Florida psychologist Julia Graber links early puberty in girls to different mental health disorders such as depressive disorders, substance use disorders, eating disorders, and disruptive behavior disorders.[37] She also stated that early puberty sets a girl up for depression in adulthood. The opposite holds for girls who mature later.

When interviewed for an article on the risks of earlier puberty in 2016, Jane Mendle of the Department of Human Development at

Cornell said, "In childhood, boys and girls have roughly the same rates of depression, but adult women are two to three times more likely to be depressed as men." Mendle continues, "That discrepancy doesn't exist at the beginning of puberty, but it is entrenched by the middle of puberty."[38]

"These kids have levels of cognitive, social and emotional development completely consistent with their age, but physically, they look older," says Mendle. "That mismatch is at the heart of the difficulties."[39]

Cultural connotations might make puberty particularly hard for girls. Being sexually mature brings specific challenges for young women, Mendle says. "In particular, there are changes in thinking of yourself as sexually desirable or physically attractive that get emphasized for girls at puberty."[40] Interestingly, the authors of the papers quoted above emphasize that the research into early puberty in boys is not being done. This is another result of the medical male gaze that blinds medical research.

Medicines prescribed for health issues during puberty fall into two categories—hormonal and psychiatric. Does being female make you more prone to disease? Certainly not. But being female has been medicalized, which is why, historically, more surgeries have been performed on women. As the medical historian Ornella Moscucci writes in her introduction to *The Science of Woman: Gynaecology and Gender in England, 1800-1929*, "A deeply entrenched belief in our culture holds that sex and reproduction are more fundamental to woman's than to man's nature. Puberty, childbirth, the menopause are deemed to affect a woman's mind and body in ways which have no counterpart in man. Because of her role in reproduction, woman is regarded as a special case, a deviation from the norm represented by the male."[41]

Medications for precocious puberty

Gonadotropin-releasing hormone analogs/agonists or GnRH analog/agonist therapy delays pubertal development. This can be in the form of a monthly injection of leuprolide acetate (Lupron Depot) or triptorelin (Trelstar and Triptodur Ki). These medications are considered the gold standard of treatment for early puberty and have been used for over 30 years.[42] The drugs inhibit physical maturation by suppressing hormone secretion. This prevents menarche and slows skeletal maturation.

These drugs have been used since the 1980s, but researchers agree that GnRH therapy retards growth and the development of sexual characteristics. There is little research into long-term effects on metabolic health and body composition. Some papers have demonstrated there is increased obesity and insulin resistance in girls taking the therapy.[43] There is also an indication that there is some decreased bone density during the time girls are taking the therapy, which could be restored after the suspension of the treatment.[44]

There had been concerns that early puberty would make shorter adults. Several papers have indicated that girls with pubertal growth spurt at 8 would be shorter than girls who went into puberty at 11. According to research, the growth spurt occurs an average of 6 to 12 months before menstruation begins. The growth spurt is triggered by steroid hormones—estradiol and testosterone— that stimulate growth hormone and IGF-1 (insulin-like growth factor).[45]

Regular menstruation usually begins 16 months after the therapy has been stopped. Infertility after the cessation of treatment has so far not been associated with GnRH analogs, but PCOS has.[46] One paper reported that PCOS occurred in 50% of the girls treated and that it occurred much younger.[47] PCOS is caused by hyperandrogenism, or high androgen hormones such as testosterone, and causes symptoms such as acne, oily skin, infertility, excess body hair, and male-pattern baldness.[48] This is a negative feedback response to suppressing gonadal production and estrogen synthesis.[49]

Because puberty involves bone growth and growth spurts, with girls having the growth spurt before boys, GnRH treatment is also used to improve adult height. There is a history of using hormones to alter an adolescent's height. A 2001 paper declares that GnRH therapy improves adult height in girls with precocious puberty.[50] It bases this conclusion on older research that associated estrogen with the fusing of growth plates and shortening of growth spurts. This paper used the Tanner stages as the basis of the criteria for normal pubertal growth in girls. The girls had precocious puberty based on breast development and estrogen levels in their bloodstream at about 6. Of the 100 girls studied, 40 had irregular periods and spotting, and 56 did not yet menstruate. It was unknown if the remaining four girls had their period or not.

They started measuring growth velocity after year two of the GnRH therapy. They concluded that the girls treated had higher growth velocity and would be taller in adulthood. What they did not mention, and what I learned from a previous paper by the same authors, is that the children in the study had precocious puberty due to adrenal tumors. A meta-analysis from 2018 found that there was little evidence that GnRH treatment increased the adult height of girls who had been treated with GnRH analogs versus girls who had not.[51]

An adolescent girl's height has been the focus of medical research since the synthesis of hormones. One paper describes the specialization of endocrinology as "fostered one of the most dynamic areas of biomedical research, establishing an important relationship between pharmaceutical research and clinical practice.[52] Another social history article describes that early endocrinology was a «combination of science, fantasy and speculation' and that research on the uses of synthetic hormones was an 'endocrinological gold rush'."[53]

The idea that tall girls should be treated with synthetic estrogen to prevent their tallness was born from the news that children with pituitary gigantism, a rare disorder in which excessive insulin-like growth factor causes tall height, had been treated with synthetic estrogen.[54] Medical treatment for tallness was more common in girls since it was not culturally accepted for girls to be tall. The treatment caused infertility and depression, "not related to adult height," as it was assumed in the 1940s that a girl who was taller than a boy would become depressed.[55] US physicians started treating girls of normal height with synthetic estrogen because girls were "becoming alarmed and unhappy about the extremes to which their exuberant, albeit normal growth was carrying them."[56]

Over the next four decades, girls in many high-income Western countries (it seemed more of a concern for middle-class parents) were treated with synthetic estrogen to keep them from getting too tall, even though the side effects were common knowledge.[57] Estrogen had been associated with the fusing of growth plates, thus preventing further growth. The clinical determination of a girl being too tall was done by estimating bone age from an x-ray of the girl's hand or wrist. The accuracy of these estimates, the basis of which was Tanner's study of English orphans in the 40s and 50s, was often disputed. Treatment was based on adult assumptions about supposed social difficulties tall girls would face and not based on any study of the psychology of the girls themselves. I mention this as a reminder that all hormone treatment is based on the assumption of male physicians about what should be suitable for women and not scientific research.

Other side effects of GnHR include:[58]

bone pain
urinary problems
hypersensitivity (itching, skin rash, fever)
gynecomastia
flushing
depression
easy and quick to anger
headache
nausea
muscle pain
joint pain
excessive sweating
fatigue
sleep disturbances

pain at the injection site
hypertension
thrombosis
vaginal spotting
pseudotumor cerebri (PTC)
headaches
papilledema
vision changes
tinnitus
anaphylactic reactions

Delayed Puberty

Delayed puberty is defined as the lack of breast development at age 13 or a year gap between breast development and menstruation. A delayed release of hormones from the pituitary gland can be a cause of delayed puberty and can be caused by a tumor in the pituitary gland. Still, hypothyroidism and adrenal deficiency, unrelated to hypopituitarism, are associated with early and delayed puberty. Both can cause delayed bone growth.

Delayed puberty happens more frequently in girls (26% in girls vs 7% in boys) due to ovarian failure. Genetic or birth abnormalities can lead to ovarian failure. This can be caused by xenoestrogens preventing proper gonadal formation in the fetus. Girls with Turner Syndrome, due to a chromosomal disorder, will be shorter in stature. Ovarian failure can also be caused by autoimmunity related to diabetes type l and type ll and Addison's disease, which is caused by tumors in the adrenal glands. These conditions are extremely rare.

Amenorrhea is the absence of menstruation. It can be transitory or permanent. It is diagnosed when there is no menstruation at the age of 13 if there has been no development of sexual characteristics or at 15 if sexual characteristics have developed. Primary amenorrhea usually involves a severe endocrine disorder, such as a tumor or malformation in the pituitary, hypothalamus, thyroid, or adrenal gland.

Secondary amenorrhea is more common and is defined as an absence of menstruation for 3 to 6 months in girls who previously had a regular period. It is usually transitory for adolescents and only an issue if the person is trying to conceive. It may bring insecurity to the teenager or her family if they think it indicates a disorder that may affect future fertility. Aside from pituitary or hypothalamic tumors, which are rare, it is associated with low thyroid function, irregular adrenal function, malnourishment, low-fat diets, and overexercise.

Amenorrhea is treated with either a selective estrogen receptor modulator (SERM), such as Clomiphene Citrate or Clomid, or synthetic estrogen therapy to force ovulation.[59] Since in the absence of a tumor in any gland involved in signaling for healthy menstruation, the cause of amenorrhea is related to a signaling or negative feedback response in some biochemical pathway in the endocrine system, overriding this negative feedback response will cause side effects.

Common side effects of Clomiphene include:[60]

headaches
mood disorders
depression
anxiety
abnormal uterine bleeding
pelvic pain
high triglycerides
hot flashes
intestinal issues
breast pain
visual disturbances
nausea
vomiting
ovarian enlargement

Polycystic Ovary Syndrome/PCOS

The rate of PCOS in adolescent females is rising dramatically. Polycystic Ovary Syndrome is the most common endocrine disorder in fertile women, but rates are increasing more in pubertal girls and adolescents than in older women.[61] It is associated with higher secretion of androgen hormones that may cause ovarian cysts, amenorrhea, infertility, and male-pattern hair growth. PCOS is seen as one of the main reasons adult women are unable to get pregnant. While recent papers have illustrated the increase in PCOS in the Middle East, China, India, and South America, the US is also seeing a significant increase in adolescent rates of PCOS.

PCOS is associated with insulin resistance metabolic disorder and an accelerated HPA axis at the beginning of puberty, specifically early adrenarche.[62] Clinical symptoms of PCOS are abdominal pain due to ovarian cysts, back pain, irregular cycles, severe acne, and even depression.[63] Studies show women with PCOS are eight times more likely to have depression than women without.[64] This is primarily because an endocrine imbalance causes PCOS, and endocrine imbalances cause depression.

Medical treatment is varied, and none of it is without side effects. Since medical treatment consists mainly of hormone replacement therapy, the following section on hormonal contraception will detail the issues with these treatments. Oral contraceptive pills and hormone replacement therapy can increase insulin resistance, weight, hair loss, bloating, acne, and depression. As is often the case with medications, treatment increases the risk of the symptoms associated with the condition treated, so in this case, treatment for PCOS can increase symptoms of PCOS.

Rates of insulin resistance are also high in PCOS. A higher BMI, higher glucose levels, and higher insulin levels make insulin resistance one of the more common characteristics of those with PCOS. I will address this further in the following chapters but mention this now to explain why medications that increase insulin sensitivity and lower blood glucose levels, such as Metformin, thiazolidinediones, Sulfonylureas, magnitudes, and incretin mimetics, are used as treatment.

Medications used to treat PCOS

Metformin reduces gluconeogenesis, intestinal absorption of carbohydrates, lipogenesis.[65]

Abdominal or stomach discomfort
cough or hoarseness
decreased appetite
diarrhea
fast or shallow breathing
fever or chills
a general feeling of discomfort
lower back or side pain
muscle pain or cramping
painful or difficult urination
sleepiness
anxiety
blurred vision
chest discomfort
cold sweats
coma
confusion
cool, pale skin
depression
difficult or labored breathing
dizziness
fast, irregular, pounding, or racing heartbeat or pulse
feeling of warmth
headache
increased hunger
increased sweating
nausea
nervousness
nightmares
redness of the face, neck, arms, and occasionally, upper chest
seizures
shakiness
slurred speech
tightness in the chest
unusual tiredness or weakness
behavior change similar to being drunk
difficulty with concentrating
drowsiness
lack or loss of strength
restless sleep

unusual sleepiness

Ploglitazone reduces fatty acid release and disrupts insulin activity. Common side effects listed by the mayoclinic.org include:[66]

chest pain
decreased urine output
dilated neck veins
extreme fatigue
irregular breathing
irregular heartbeat
problems with teeth
swelling of the face, fingers, feet, or lower legs
tightness in the chest
trouble breathing
weight gain
pain or swelling in the arms or legs without an injury
pale skin
swelling
trouble with breathing when active
unusual bleeding or bruising
unusual tiredness or weakness
dark urine
loss of appetite
nausea or vomiting
stomach pain
unexplained, rapid weight gain
yellow eyes or skin

Due to increased reports of bladder cancer, it has been withdrawn from the French market. The US FDA added a black box warning due to the cancer risk, but the sale of the medication has not been suspended.[67]

Rosiglitazone increases cellular insulin sensitivity. Common side effects listed by the mayoclinic.org include:[68]

abdominal or stomach pain
blurred vision
chest pain or discomfort
decrease in the amount of urine
dry mouth
flushed, dry skin
fruit-like breath odor
increased hunger

increased thirst
increased urination
irregular heartbeat
nausea
noisy, rattling breathing
pain in the shoulders, arms, jaw, or neck
pale skin
rapid or unusual weight gain
sweating
swelling of the fingers, hands, feet, or lower legs
trouble breathing
unexplained weight loss
unusual bleeding or bruising
unusual tiredness or weakness
vomiting
anxiety
chills
cold sweats
coma
confusion
dark urine
depression
dizziness
fast heartbeat
headache
loss of appetite
nightmares
seizures
shakiness
slurred speech
blue lips and fingernails
changes in vision
coughing that sometimes produces a pink, frothy sputum
hive-like swelling on the face, eyelids, lips, tongue, throat, hands, legs, feet, or sex organs
itching or skin rash
light-colored stools
redness of the skin
yellow eyes or skin

Due to its association with increased heart disease, Rosiglitazone has been banned in India.[69]

Liraglutide increases insulin secretion.[70]

Common side effects listed by the mayoclinic.org include:

peripheral edema
bladder pain
bloody or cloudy urine
chills
cough
diarrhea
difficult, burning, or painful urination
fever
frequent urge to urinate
general feeling of discomfort or illness
headache
hoarseness
joint pain
loss of appetite
lower back or side pain
muscle aches and pains
nausea
runny nose
shivering
sore throat
sweating
trouble sleeping
unusual tiredness or weakness
vomiting
blurred vision
dizziness
nervousness
pounding in the ears
slow or fast heartbeat
anxiety
cold sweats
confusion
cool, pale skin
depression
hives or welts, itching, or skin rash
increased hunger
large, hive-like swelling on the face, eyelids, lips, tongue, throat, hands, legs, feet, or genitals
loss of consciousness
nightmares
redness of the skin

seizures
shakiness
slurred speech
agitation
clay-colored stools
confusion
dark urine
decreased awareness or responsiveness
decreased urine output
depression
difficulty with swallowing
hostility
irritability
muscle twitching
puffiness or swelling of the eyelids or around the eyes, face, lips, or tongue
rapid weight gain
severe sleepiness
swelling of the face, ankles, or hands
tightness in the chest
unpleasant breath odor
vomiting of blood
yellow eyes or skin

Exenatide

Common side effects listed by the mayoclinic.org include:[71]

nausea
vomiting
diarrhea
constipation
decreased appetite
jittery feeling
dizziness
heartburn
headache
weakness
sweating
ongoing pain that begins in the upper left or middle of the stomach but may spread to the back with or without vomiting
hives
rash
itching
swelling of the face, throat, tongue, lips, or eyes
dizziness or fainting
rapid heartbeat

difficulty breathing or swallowing
injection-site pain, swelling, blisters, itching, or nodules
pain in the right or upper middle stomach area, nausea, vomiting, fever, or yellowing of skin or eyes
changes in the color or amount of urine
urinating more or less often than usual
swelling of the arms, hands, feet, ankles, or lower legs
unusual bleeding or bruising

Semaglutide increases insulin secretion inhibits glucagon release and suppresses hepatic gluconeogenesis.
Common side effects listed by the mayoclinic.org include:[72]

diarrhea
constipation
hair loss
belching
bloated, full feeling
excess air or gas in the stomach or intestines
gaseous stomach pain
heartburn
passing gas
recurrent fever
stomach discomfort, fullness, or pain
yellow eyes or skin
burning feeling in the chest or stomach
indigestion
stomach upset
tenderness in the stomach area
anxiety
blurred vision
chest tightness
chills
cold sweats
confusion
cool, pale skin
cough
darkened urine
difficulty swallowing
discouragement
dizziness
fast heartbeat
feeling sad or empty
headache
hives, itching

increased heart rate
increased hunger
irritability
lack of appetite
large, hive-like swelling on the face, eyelids, lips, tongue, throat, hands, legs, feet, or sex organs
loss of consciousness
loss of interest or pleasure
nausea
nightmares
pains in stomach, side, or abdomen, possibly radiating to the back
puffiness or swelling of the eyelids or around the eyes, face, lips, or tongue
redness of the skin
seizures
shakiness
skin rash
slurred speech
tiredness
trouble breathing
trouble concentrating
trouble sleeping
unusual tiredness or weakness
vomiting

Sitagliptin increases insulin production and decreases hepatic glucose overproduction

Common side effects listed by the mayoclinic.org include:[73]

anxiety
blurred vision
chills
cold sweats
confusion
cool, pale skin
depression
dizziness
fast heartbeat
headache
increased hunger
loss of consciousness
nausea
nightmares
seizures
shakiness
slurred speech

unusual tiredness or weakness
blistering, peeling, loosening of the skin
diarrhea
hives or welts, itching, or skin rash
hive-like swelling on the face, eyelids, lips, tongue, throat, hands, legs, feet, or sex organs
loss of appetite
pains in the stomach, side, or abdomen, possibly radiating to the back
puffiness or swelling of the eyelids or around the eyes, face, lips, or tongue
red skin lesions, often with a purple center
redness of the skin
severe joint pain
sores, ulcers, or white spots in the mouth or on the lips
vomiting
body aches or pain
cough
difficulty with breathing
ear congestion
fever
loss of voice
muscle aches
sneezing
sore throat
stuffy or runny nose
diarrhea
stomach pain

Dapagliflozin blocks glucose reabsorption in the kidney, increasing urinary glucose excretion and reducing blood glucose levels. Common side effects listed by the mayoclinic.org include:[74]

anxiety
bladder pain
bloody or cloudy urine
blurred vision
chills
cold sweats
confusion
cool, pale skin
decreased frequency or amount of urine
depression
difficult, burning, or painful urination
dizziness
fast heartbeat
frequent urge to urinate

headache
increased hunger
increased thirst
itching of the vagina or genitals
loss of appetite
loss of consciousness
lower back or side pain
nausea
nightmares
seizures
shakiness
slurred speech
swelling of the face, fingers, or lower legs
thick, white vaginal discharge with mild or no odor
trouble breathing
unusual tiredness or weakness
vomiting
foul-smelling discharge from the penis
pain in the skin around the penis
rash of the penis
redness, itching, or swelling of the penis
cough
difficulty with swallowing
dizziness, faintness, or lightheadedness when getting up suddenly from a lying or sitting position
dry mouth
fainting
increase in heart rate
hive-like swelling on the face, eyelids, lips, tongue, throat, hands, legs, feet, or genitals
lightheadedness
puffiness or swelling of the eyelids or around the eyes, face, lips, or tongue
rapid breathing
skin rash, hives, or itching
sunken eyes
sweating
tightness in the chest
wrinkled skin
fever
flushed, dry skin
fruit-like breath odor
loss of consciousness

pain, tenderness, redness, or swelling of the area between the anus and genitals
stomach pain
unexplained weight loss
muscle aches
sore throat
stuffy or runny nose
back pain
difficulty having a bowel movement
pain in the arms or legs

Empagliflozin blocks glucose reabsorption in the kidney, increasing urinary glucose excretion and reducing blood glucose levels.[75] Common side effects listed by the mayoclinic.org include:

bladder pain
bloody or cloudy urine
change in the color, amount, or odor of vaginal discharge
difficult, burning, or painful urination
frequent urge to urinate
itching, stinging, or redness of the vaginal area
lower back or side pain
pain during sexual intercourse
discharge with a strong odor from the penis
increased volume of pale, dilute urine
redness, itching, swelling, or pain around the penis
waking to urinate at night
anxiety
blurred vision
chills
cold sweats
confusion
decreased urination
dizziness, faintness, or lightheadedness when getting up suddenly from a lying or sitting position
fast heartbeat
headache
increased hunger
nausea
nightmares
rapid breathing
seizures
shakiness
slurred speech
sweating

unusual tiredness or weakness
dry mouth
fever
flushed, dry skin
fruit-like breath odor
increased thirst
itching, skin rash
large, hive-like swelling on the face, eyelids, lips, tongue, throat, hands, legs, feet, or genitals
loss of appetite
loss of consciousness
pain, tenderness, redness, or swelling of the area between the anus and genitals
redness of the skin
stomach pain
sunken eyes
trouble breathing
unexplained weight loss
vomiting
weight gain
wrinkled skin
body aches or pain
cough
loss of voice
muscle pain or stiffness
runny or stuffy nose
sneezing

Liagliptin increases the production of insulin and decreases the production of glucagon by the pancreas.
Common side effects listed by the mayoclinic.org include:[76]

anxiety
blurred vision
chills
cold sweats
confusion
cool, pale skin
depression
dizziness
fast heartbeat
headache
increased hunger
loss of consciousness
nausea

nightmares
seizures
shakiness
slurred speech
unusual tiredness or weakness
bloating
constipation
cough
fever
hives, welts, itching, or skin rash
large, hard skin blisters
large, hive-like swelling on the face, eyelids, lips, tongue, throat, hands, legs, feet, or sex organs
loss of appetite
pains in the stomach, side, or abdomen, possibly radiating to the back
puffiness or swelling of the eyelids or around the eyes, face, lips, or tongue
redness of the skin
severe joint pain
muscle aches
sore throat
stuffy or runny nose
diarrhea

Canagliflozin increases glucose excretion in the urine by reducing the re-absorption of filtered glucose. Common side effects listed by mayoclinic.org include:[77]

bladder pain
bloating
bloody or cloudy urine
decreased frequency or amount of urine
difficult, burning, or painful urination
discharge with a strong odor from the penis
frequent urge to urinate
increased thirst
increased urge to urinate during the night
indigestion
itching of the vagina or outside of the genitals
loss of appetite
lower back or side pain
nausea
pain during sexual intercourse
pain in the skin around the penis
problems in urination or an increase in the amount of urine
redness, itching, or swelling of the penis

swelling of the face, fingers, or lower legs
thick, white vaginal discharge with mild or no odor
trouble breathing
unusual tiredness or weakness
vomiting
waking to urinate at night
weight gain
anxiety
blurred vision
chills
cold sweats
confusion
cool, pale skin
depression
dizziness
dry mouth
fast or irregular heartbeat
flushing, redness of the skin
headache
hives or welts, itching skin, rash
increased hunger
itching skin
hive-like swelling on the face, eyelids, lips, tongue, throat, hands, legs, feet, or genitals
nightmares
redness of the skin
seizures
shakiness
slurred speech
hot skin
dizziness, faintness, or lightheadedness when getting up suddenly from a lying or sitting position
fever
flushed, dry skin
frequent or painful urination
fruit-like breath odor
increased urination
loss of consciousness
numbness or tingling in the hands, feet, or lips
pain, tenderness, redness, or swelling of the area between the anus and genitals
stomach pain
sweating

unexplained weight loss
weakness or heaviness of the legs
yellow eyes or skin

Corticosteroids are also used to treat PCOS. Some studies have shown that prednisone and dexamethasone can trigger ovulation. Prednisone sold as Rayos, Deltasone, Prednidot, Prednisone Intensol, Steraped, and Steraped DS, and dexamethasone, sold as Decadron, Dexamethasone Intensol, Dexasone, Solurex, and Baycadro, can reduce adrenal androgens on follicular growth simply because it blocks natural adrenal hormone synthesis. This is short-lived, however, because dexamethasone and prednisone raise adrenal hormone levels. Synthetic cortisone, the wonder drug of the 1940s, causes horrible side effects, and prolonged use is never encouraged.

Prednisone
Common side effects listed by mayoclinic.org include:[78]

edema
muscle weakness
bloating
thin skin
sweating
thin skin
excitement
changes in menstrual bleeding
confusion
restlessness
nausea or vomiting
acne
moon face
weight gain
headache
heart problems
depression
insomnia
low potassium
high blood pressure
anxiety
infection
osteoporosis
stomach ulcers

insulin resistance and diabetes
cataracts
glaucoma
allergic reaction

Dexamethasone
Common side effects listed by mayoclinic.org include:[79]

aggression
agitation
anxiety
blurred vision
decrease in the amount of urine
dizziness
fast, slow, pounding, or irregular heartbeat or pulse
headache
irritability
mental depression
mood changes
nervousness
noisy, rattling breathing
numbness or tingling in the arms or legs
pounding in the ears
swelling of the fingers, hands, feet, or lower legs
trouble thinking, speaking, or walking
troubled breathing at rest
weight gain
abdominal or stomach cramping backache
bloody, black, or tarry stools
cough or hoarseness
darkening of the skin
decrease in height
decreased vision
diarrhea
dry mouth
eye pain
eye tearing
facial hair growth in females
fainting
fatigue
fever or chills
flushed, dry skin
fractures
fruit-like breath odor
full or round face, neck, or trunk

heartburn and/or indigestion
increased hunger
increased thirst
increased urination
loss of appetite
loss of sexual desire or ability
lower back or side pain
menstrual irregularities
muscle pain or tenderness
muscle wasting or weakness
nausea
pain in the back, ribs, arms, or legs
painful or difficult urination
skin rash
sleeplessness
sweating
trouble healing
trouble sleeping
unexplained weight loss
unusual tiredness or weakness
vision changes
vomiting

Gonadotrophins-synthetic FSH, synthetic LH, and synthetic hCG are also used to treat PCOS, and I have explained their side effects above.

Endometriosis

Endometriosis was commonly associated with adult women. In the last decade, scientists have demonstrated an increased rate of endometriosis in young girls with symptoms such as pelvic pain and dysmenorrhea. The lesions seen in adolescent girls can be more painful than those in adult women. Endometriosis is associated with dysregulated estrogen secretion. The medications used in treatment are oral contraceptives, GnRH analogs/agonists, anti-inflammatory pain-killers, synthetic progesterone.

Birth Control Pills or Other Types of Hormonal Medication

As of 2022, the most common oral contraceptive pills are Diane, Brenda, Juliet, Estelle, Yasmin, and Valette. The synthetic hormonal ingredients in combined oral contraceptives are ethinylestradiol, desogestrel, and gestone. Synthetic progesterone-only contraceptive drugs are made of progestin and are sold as Provera, Prometrium, and Aygestin.

What is the problem with synthetic estrogen? Estrogen promotes cell growth. Synthetic estrogen is not entirely converted in the human body, and excess estrogen accumulates in tissues with receptors for it. It stimulates tumor growth in the breasts and uterus. All the scientists involved with the development saw this result in their animal lab tests. Synthetic estrogen is many times stronger than the estrogen produced in the human body.

In 1932, Antoine Lacassagne gave Butenandt's estrogen to mice and made them have mammary cancer. In 1939, the *Journal of the American Medical Association* published an editorial against estrogen therapy, saying, "The possibility of carcinoma cannot be ignored. It appears likely that the medical profession may be importuned to prescribe patients large doses of high potency estrogens, such as stilbestrol, because of the ease of administration of these products."[80] The authors emphasized the importance of prescribing estrogen therapy for a short time and that the use should be gradually tapered off. Since the invention of the pill, many girls have been prescribed synthetic estrogen in their birth control pills from the day they start menstruating until they reach menopause to prevent pregnancy, even though other non-hormonal barrier birth control methods are just as effective. Girls prescribed the pill only stop taking them or other forms of hormonal birth control if they choose to get pregnant.

The first synthetic birth control invented was DES, diethylstilbestrol. Following the drug companies' huge marketing campaign, DES was approved in 1941, although it was already clear by 1940 that DES caused cancer. Cancer researcher Dr. Michael Boris Shimkin, who later linked smoking to lung cancer, published an article in the *Journal of the National Cancer Institute* describing how DES spontaneously produced breast cancer in female mice.[81]

Ethinyl estradiol was first synthesized in 1938 by Hans Herloff Inhoffen and Walter Hohlweg at Schering, a German pharmaceutical company. Charles Dodds had synthesized DES in England. There had been a race as to who could come up with the first synthetic estrogen. Since there was a war on, DES was first used in the US and the UK. Ethinyl estradiol (EE) has a potency 500 times more than 17- estradiol, the natural estrogen produced in the human body.[82] Proponents of birth control pills claim that EE is much less potent than DES. This is not true. In a study that compared the potency of natural estrogen and synthetic estrogen's ability to bind to estrogen receptors,

DES was 1.1 times more potent in these receptor binding assays than E2, while EE2 was slightly less potent than E2.[83]

Birth control pills cause breast, uterine, and cervical cancer, but the sale of estrogen has always been lucrative for pharmaceutical companies and doctors. In the 1930s and 40s, the research that demonstrated estrogens could cause cancer had only been seen in mice and rats. Proponents of hormone therapy did not believe—or did not want to believe—that it would have the same carcinogenic effect on women. Reports would take two decades to surface that women taking these estrogens were getting cancer.[84]

Biochemists had worked feverishly to isolate reproductive hormones, and in the 1950s, pharmaceutical companies in Canada, the US, and Germany were creating massive campaigns to market their products to menopausal women. Surgeons had marketed hysterectomies and oophorectomies in the nineteenth century when industrial England saw a surge in cervical cancer.

Cancer was seen as a stigma and was already discussed as a genetic trait. Women had preventative surgery to ensure they did not get it—just as a woman today sometimes has mastectomies if they have a gene that is reportedly supposed to predispose them to breast cancer. Just as invasive and ineffective surgeries became a societal obligation for women, marketing menopause as a deficiency created a market for new products.

Since estrogen was linked to fertility, menopause, by consequence, meant women were deficient in it. Estrogen was isolated, but it was not yet measured. Since fertility meant, to men, health and beauty, a decline in the hormone that signified fertility would hasten the arrival of all the physical changes associated with aging. They did not yet understand that other organs and peripheral tissue take over estrogen production during menopause. This was not discovered until 1988.[85] In 1960, the FDA approved the sale of Enovid 10, which was the world's first pharmaceutical birth control pill.

It was from Butenandt's work that ethinyl estradiol (EE), a synthetic steroidal estrogen, was synthesized. There are three kinds of estrogens produced in the female body: estrone (E1), which is prevalent in females before puberty and after menopause; estradiol (E2), which is the estrogen produced in the ovaries when women begin menstruating and are not pregnant, and estriol (E3), which is primarily produced during pregnancy.

Ethinyl estradiol was approved for use in the United States in 1949 and is still a component of modern birth control pills. Ethinyl estradiol was marketed as both a contraceptive and a treatment for menopausal symptoms. However, it was eventually removed from this latter market and repackaged as a combined estrogen and progesterone because of the reports of unopposed estrogen and increased endometrial cancer. EE also has side effects like breast tenderness, bloating, nausea, headache, and weight gain. Women who took ethinyl estradol products also experienced a greater risk of blood clots and venous thromboembolism. Butenandt also warned about the possibility that the hormones could cause cancer.

In 1953, Schering Pharmaceuticals (now Bayer Schering Pharma AG) released a video to "educate" physicians and promote ethinyl estradiol therapy—which is still the primary component in contraceptives today. It opens to a matronly woman, somewhere in the country, taking in laundry from the backyard, while the male voiceover states that declining reproductive capacity only happens to women. We presume this "country woman" is eating a healthy diet and breathing fresh country air and is engaged only in "housework." Just as the voiceover has finished saying, "While the majority of women pass through this change without problems," [women in the country] the film cuts to a busy doctor's office where several smartly dressed younger women wait their turn. The voiceover explains their presence by saying, "The menopause can bring symptoms so disturbing that medical help must be sought" and that "this can occur as young as 35" the man's voice explains. The final image is of a doctor prescribing ethinyl estradiol, as the voiceover concludes, "Woman's menopausal symptoms are caused by her emotional fragility, and can only be helped, must be helped by sedatives and estrogens."[86]

Symptoms Associated with the Pill

Blood clotting—the pill causes changes in how blood clots. Increased clotting factors can cause deep vein thrombosis, pulmonary thrombosis, heart attacks, and strokes. The pill is associated with blood clotting because it reduces blood velocity in circulation and increases blood coagulation. "Pill users form blood clots faster than non-users, and the clots they form are firmer. The pill increases the odds that the veins may become varicose in time." wrote Barbara Seaman in her book *The Doctors' Case Against the Pill*. Blood clots can form in any veins—brain, legs, arms, lungs, heart, etc.[87]

Heart disease—the pill changes metabolism. It raises blood pressure, increases insulin resistance, and changes how glucose, lipids, proteins, and minerals such as magnesium are metabolized.

Many researchers have tried to place the blame on the increased atherosclerosis risk found in women who take the pill on the women who also smoke. Both smoking and oral contraceptives increase the risk of heart disease. After factoring smoking, age, and economic status, a study from 1979 concluded that women who took the pill were still two times as likely to die from vascular diseases than women who did not.[88]

Stroke—It could start as a headache. It may be pain behind the eyes, dizziness, impaired vision, neck pain, or numbness in your face, arms, or legs. These are some of the many symptoms that warn of a blood clot in the brain or an ischemic stroke. Papers on this danger have been published since 1968, but a meta-analysis from 2000 underlined that the risk is ever-present in those taking the pill.[89]

Cancer—Synthetic estrogens and progesterones have been associated with cancer in all tissues since they were first invented. A meta-analysis from 2020 warned that the pill, be it either a combination of the synthetic ethinyl estradiol or progestin, undoubtedly increased the risk of cervical cancer.[90]

Diabetes—Oral contraceptives cause insulin resistance because synthetic hormones affect glucose metabolism, be it from the foods you eat or the sugar naturally made in the liver. This is primarily because both synthetic estrogen and progesterone raise cortisol levels.[91]

Women are advised to take oral contraceptives with low amounts of either to minimize their risk of diabetes. Why take any risk at all? Dr. V. Wynn's papers spanned decades and summarized the issue succinctly. Dr. V. Wynn, a British physician who regularly criticized the standard prescription of the birth control pill, was concerned that the insulin resistance the pill caused would not be diagnosed, especially in younger women, because they were not adequately tested for glucose tolerance.[92]

Kraft's five-hour glucose tolerance test has been accepted as the best way to diagnose insulin resistance and hyperinsulinemia. This is still not the gold standard for diagnosing pre-diabetes, although it should be. It takes more time, so the fasting glucose test is the test that is regularly conducted.

"The machinery of metabolism is beautifully complex and harmonious. It is easy enough to dominate it by introducing substances like the synthetic hormones in the Pill," he instructed his students. "But we have no idea of what risks we run by assuming control of such a delicate process. After all, there is no cell in the body that is not affected by oral contraceptives—nerve cells, skin cells, liver cells, blood cells."[93]

The pill affects sex drive and orgasm—this would be primarily because it raises cortisol levels. It can cause sterility, genetic changes, jaundice, low thyroid function, weight gain, and UTIs. It can cause skin and gum problems and depression.

All steroid hormones affect brain chemistry. Estrogen and progesterone influence levels of important mood-stabilizing neurotransmitters GABA, serotonin, adrenalin, and dopamine. Both progesterone modulate these neurotransmitters. Recent papers have outlined the dangers of both synthetic estrogen and progesterone, the ingredients of oral contraceptives. One demonstrated that these effects were not limited to oral contraceptives but also associated with synthetic progesterone levonorgestrel common in IUDs. Women with hormonal IUDs that had progesterone had higher levels of anxiety, depression, and sleep issues.

Higher levels of depression have been linked to women who use the pill since 1969. British researchers documented that the suicide rate was two to three times higher in women who took the pill and that one out of three women taking the pill studied showed signs of depression.[94] They also saw that pill users were deficient in vitamin B6, which is essential to brain health.

A 2016 Danish study published in the *JAMA Psychology Journal* reported that women using hormonal birth control were more likely to use antidepressants.[95] This is particularly frightening because national health services in European communities push the birth control pill on teenage girls, just as they push hormone therapy on middle-aged women and antidepressants on women past sixty. What is even more frightening is that in 1969, Harold Williams published *Pregnant or Dead* and included statistics of the spike in suicide rates in young women taking the pill.[96]

Papers from 2022 and 2023 are sounding the same alarm. One study of 900,000 women found that oral contraceptives were linked to higher rates of adolescent girls taking anti-depressants.[97] Women taking the pill concluded that girls who began to use combined synthetic estrogen and progesterone contraceptive pills as teenagers had a 130% higher incidence of symptoms of depression. In adult users, it was progestin-only contraceptives that increased rates of depression by 92%. Each paper concludes by recommending that doctors carefully screen women before prescribing hormonal contraceptives. Is this being done? Nevertheless, why take drugs associated with these terrible side effects when there are barrier methods that have none?

Thyroid Function

Hormonal contraceptives alter thyroid function. Synthetic estrogens increase the protein that binds to thyroid hormones in the bloodstream by 50%, thus reducing the reserve of thyroid hormone in the bloodstream essential for all cells in the human body. The increased thyroid-binding proteins gobble up the thyroid hormones and make them useless. Hypothyroid women who take the pill need up to 45% more thyroid hormone medication. This would mean that the thyroid levels of women who have not been diagnosed with thyroid issues and are not taking any thyroid hormone would need that much more if they take the pill. Combined with the fact that adolescents require 40% more thyroid hormone during puberty to build sexual characteristics, the pill renders them hypothyroid. The pill also changes the results of thyroid blood tests results and will show higher levels of free 4 and lower TSH results, which will prevent females from being diagnosed as hypothyroid.[98]

Hormonal contraceptives raise levels of inflammation in the body and contribute to autoimmunity This increases the risks of Crohn's disease, Lupus, and interstitial cystitis. Progesterone-only contraceptives increased dermatitis, eczema, alopecia, acne, and urticaria. A paper from 2010 studying why, after decades of lower rates of rheumatoid arthritis, rates started skyrocketing from 1995 to 2007 and concluded that more women taking the pill were to blame. While one paper explained how synthetic estrogen was inflammatory, another said the same about synthetic progesterone, commonly found in IUDs.[99]

Oral contraceptives increase the risk of liver cancer by two to three times. Jaundice is considered a common side effect of taking the pill. The rate of hepatic adenomas increases the longer a woman takes the pills. A woman who takes oral contraceptives for 109 months has a 25 times higher risk of developing liver tumors than one who takes the pill for 12 months. Suspending the pill makes the liver tumors disappear.[100] One paper showed that 70% of women were admitted for cholecystectomies because synthetic estrogen changes the flow and composition of bile. The oral contraceptives also cause gallstones.[101] While the risk of gallbladder disease is higher in women who take the pill at all ages, it is remarkably higher in young women who take the pill and can occur rapidly as soon as younger women begin to take it.

The pill will prevent the metabolism of essential nutrients, specifically vitamins B6 and 12, vitamin C, and trace minerals such as zinc, which will cause malnourishment. The lower zinc levels associated with taking the pill are primarily because it increases copper levels, which will oppose zinc. I will explain how malnourishment causes the health issues that can come with puberty in the first place. Still, it is crucial to realize that taking the pill for the issues caused by a hormonal imbalance in the first place causes malnourishment and only worsens both of the causative factors. Barrier methods to prevent pregnancy don't have any side effects.

Besides synthetic hormonal drugs, the symptoms associated with the perils of puberty are addressed with psychiatric medications. Antidepressants don't work. They increase ideas of suicidal ideation. Several studies I cited earlier make that clear. They all work on the same pathway, the GABA system. There is no proof that SSRIs work better than placebos to treat depression. They numb you. Over time, the body will respond to any suppression with a negative feedback response; whatever caused the anxiety or depression will worsen because antidepressants cause an up-regulation in GABA receptor expression. This amplification eventually burns out the GABA receptors and causes an increase in glutamate, the excitatory neurotransmitter, which causes more anxiety.

A Harvard paper in 2018 was shocked to announce that antidepressant use had increased by 400% from 1994 to 2008.[102] It also said that females were 2.5 times more likely to be prescribed antidepressants at ages as low as 12. It is less likely that what today is considered mental health problems would be treated with surgery today, as they were until the 1920s; sedatives have become the gold standard to treat emotional disturbances. Hostility, anger, aggression, and panic attacks are associated with the use of anti-depressants. A 2015 study concluded those taking antidepressants were "much more likely" to commit suicide.[103] As with any drug, side effects depend on which one you take. Cymbalta has been linked to liver failure, Zoloft to diarrhea, Effexor to suicide, high blood pressure, and gastrointestinal bleeding.

Antidepressants

Common side effects listed by the mayoclinic.org include:[104]

nausea
depression
tremors
bladder problems
low thyroid hormone levels
anxiety
restlessness
decreased sex drive
dizziness
weight gain
weight loss
sweating
insomnia
fatigue
dry mouth
diarrhea
constipation
headaches

Gabapentin, regularly prescribed to adults for neuropathy and epilepsy and off-label for insomnia, is being prescribed to teenagers for anxiety and social phobia.

Common side effects of Gabapentin as listed by mayoclinic.org:[105]

dizziness
drowsiness
weakness
fatigue
nausea
diarrhea
constipation
blurred vision
headache
breast swelling
dry mouth
loss of balance or coordination.

Anti-anxiety drugs often are benzodiazepines, such as Xanax. There is a disturbing trend in the increase of prescriptions of benzodiazepines in children documented by research papers describing the increase in the United States, the United Kingdom, and Ireland for anxiety, insomnia, concentration, and behavioral issues. Some papers describe an increase in children prescribed benzodiazepines and children who find them in their parent's medicine cabinet, using benzodiazepines as recreational drugs. Since Heather Ashton's work in the 1980s, it has been known that long-term benzodiazepine use can have lifelong consequences and that suspending or tapering the medication comes with terrible symptoms. That they should never be prescribed for more than two weeks should be common medical knowledge, but they are often prescribed for longer periods of time, which can lead to abuse, as they are so difficult to come off of.

Common side effects listed by the mayoclinic.org include:[106]

nausea
vomiting
diarrhea
headache
drowsiness
dry mouth
insomnia
nervousness, agitation or restlessness
dizziness
sexual problems, such as reduced sexual desire, difficulty reaching orgasm
impact on appetite, leading to weight loss or weight gain
confusion
stomach upset
headaches
dizziness
seizures
trouble concentrating
poor coordination
decreased appetite
dry mouth
slurred speech
blurred vision
constipation
depression
diarrhea
hives
irritability
swelling in your hands or feet

weak and rapid heartbeat
abdominal cramps
hallucinations
irregular menstrual cycle
tolerance
withdrawal effects

Attention Deficit Disorder, now called Attention Deficit Hyperactive Disorder

In the last decades, scientists bemoaned that girls were not adequately diagnosed with ADHD. Doctors in both the US and Sweden studied the skyrocketing diagnoses. Subsequent medication of children were possibly due to a "family spillover effect" when younger siblings and cousins of children who had been diagnosed with ADHD were given the same diagnosis since ADHD is believed to be a genetic disorder. Researchers of two papers concluded that children were being medicated for ADHD when they possibly should not be.[107] Simultaneously, scientists were concerned that girls were under the radar. Why weren't they being diagnosed at the same rate as male children?[108]

A paper published in 2014 claimed to have the answer.[109] Girls' hormones were different because it's different for girls! Just as a menopausal woman is supposedly in danger of cognitive decline due to the assumption that there is a decline in estrogen (there is not a decline in estrogen. The adrenal glands keep synthesizing estrogen just fine), a girl with a period may be unable to pay attention at school because estrogen declines during menstruation. She may be grumpy and moody and cry. That's what a website called yourcycle.org is telling girls. Because, you know, females are more emotional. This is what science has been telling women since Hippocrates. It has become common to prescribe pre-teen girls birth control not to prevent pregnancy (they are too young to have sex and may not have their cycle yet, but they do have puberty), but to treat symptoms of ADHD.

The problem with this is that papers are now raising the alarm that girls prescribed birth control to control their ADHD symptoms had higher rates of depression than girls who took amphetamines to control their symptoms. I don't agree with the amphetamines either, but I'm trying to illustrate how females are treated differently by the medical establishment based on what I call the male medical gaze.

What is interesting is that the girls who are diagnosed with ADHD are prescribed synthetic estrogen because they have antisocial, hostile, and adversarial behavior and because they have a cycle and boys don't. The claim that estrogen increases dopamine and serotonin levels is the same argument that is given to women who feel depressed or volatile when their estrogen levels reduce with menopause. We know since Labrie's revelation in the 1980s that women's estrogen levels do not reduce because adrenal synthesis keeps making estrogens. The ovarian production of estradiol reduces simply because women do not evolve to have children after their 50s. There is plenty of estrogen in the form of estrone after menopause.

The reason why girls in the mid-19th century were given sedatives and subjected to surgeries before hormones had been discovered was girls who reached puberty were described as antisocial, hostile, and given to adversarial behavior, in the sense that they questioned what their parents told them to do. The Victorian era expected demure and silent girls who followed their mother's example in growing into a womanhood that would ensure their eligibility as wives. Since doctors claimed that their nerves were weakened by menstruation, they were in danger of emotional volatility, a morbid imagination, fits of rage, and fatigue, but also silly, vain, and easily given to depravity. Lasègue's 1873 paper "De l'Anorexie Hystérique" described selfish and vain girls who ruined family life. He wrote that hysterical girls "do not forgive, and, considering that hostilities have begun, they grant themselves the right to continue them with a relentless tenacity."[110]

Girls as young as 9 are prescribed hormone replacement therapy. Girls and their parents are told the pill will improve symptoms that can come during puberty in the presence of a hormonal imbalance. They are not prescribed the pill as a means of birth control. They are told it will prevent acne. With the recent phenomenon of plummeting ages of puberty, that means more and more girls are being subjected to the possible side effects of synthetic hormones scientists have known about since the beginning. Furthermore, the chance of severe side effects illustrated above is increased the longer the person takes the synthetic hormones.

Body Odor/Sweating

The increase of androgen hormones that comes with adrenarche during puberty will cause body odor and be abnormal if the steroid hormones are out of balance. The primary androgen is cortisol, which is part of the physiological stress response. We know that fear has an odor and that fear causes sweating because the stress response causes a vasomotor reaction that comes with increased body temperature. The medical response to this is that bacterial overgrowth is involved. Every mucus-bearing tissue on the body has bacteria that protect the organism from pathogens. This means that underarm and vaginal tissue has a great deal of good bacteria. This presence of this bacteria is also a huge market for products that will mask any odor at all. Not only are deodorants often full of dangerous chemicals, but they also disrupt the balance of the necessary bacteria. This is what leads to bacterial overgrowth. Vulval tissue is exceptionally sensitive to chemicals that block the apocrine glands of these tissues. Candida is the most common result of bacterial overgrowth. What candida loves is sugar, both the sugar from the diet, but also the sugar that is produced by the liver during a stress response.

A 2002 paper sought to test the scent fear and found that cortisol levels were higher than they usually would have been at the time of day when the women in the experiment were shown a scary movie.[111] They also concluded that the women participating found that the underarm pads that became sweaty when they watched the movie smelled much stronger and malodorous than those who did not. The pads worn during the scary movie smelled unpleasant and like aggression. The increase of adrenal hormones, including cortisol, is part of an imbalance.

Drugs and other substances Interfering with Thyroid Function can also cause acne. These are the medications commonly used to treat acne.

Tretinoin is a retinol, so the side effects are related to Vitamin A toxicity. Retinol products also cause central hypothyroidism. Common side effects listed by the mayoclinic.org include:[112]

pale skin
skin irritation
bone swelling
crusty skin
fever
headache
hives
anxiety
bone pain
burning
diarrhea
discomfort or pain in chest
blistering
bloody stools
blue lips and fingernails
blurred vision
hair loss
indigestion
pain surrounding the treated areas
peeling or flaky skin
bleeding
clumsiness or unsteadiness when walking
difficulty in moving
teratogenic, so can cause birth defects.

The antiseptic benzoyl peroxide is used to treat acne.
Common side effects listed by the mayoclinic.org include:[113]

chest tightness
cough
difficulty swallowing
dizziness
fainting
fast heartbeat
hives, itching, or skin rash
increased sensitivity of the skin to sunlight
large, hive-like swelling on face, eyelids, lips, tongue, throat, hands, legs, feet, or sex organs
redness or other discoloration of the skin
severe sunburn
swelling of the eyes, face, lips, or tongue
tightness in the throat
trouble breathing
unusual tiredness or weakness
dryness or peeling of the skin (may occur after a few days)
feeling of warmth, mild stinging, and redness of the skin

The antibiotic Clindamycin is used to treat acne.
Common side effects listed by the mayoclinic.org include:[114]

abdominal or stomach cramps, pain, or tenderness
black, tarry stools
bleeding gums
blistering, peeling, or loosening of the skin
bloating
blood in the urine or stools
blurred vision
chest pain
chills
clay-colored stools
cloudy urine
confusion
cough or hoarseness
dark urine
decrease in the amount of urine
diarrhea
diarrhea, watery and severe, which may also be bloody
difficulty with swallowing
dizziness
dizziness, faintness, or lightheadedness

dry mouth
fast heartbeat
fever with or without chills
general feeling of tiredness or weakness
headache
heartburn
heart stops
hives or welts, itching, or skin rash
increased thirst
itching of the vagina or genital area
joint or muscle pain
loss of appetite
lower back or side pain
nausea or vomiting
no breathing
no pulse or blood pressure
pain during sexual intercourse
pain in the lower back or side
painful or difficult urination
pinpoint red spots on the skin
puffiness or swelling of the eyelids or around the eyes, face, lips, or tongue
rash with flat lesions or small raised lesions on the skin
red skin lesions, often with a purple center
red, irritated eyes
redness of the skin
sore throat
sores, ulcers, or white spots in the mouth or on the lips
swollen glands
thick, white vaginal discharge with no odor or with a mild odor
thirst
tightness in the chest
trouble breathing
unconscious
unpleasant breath odor
unusual bleeding or bruising
unusual tiredness or weakness
unusual weight loss
vomiting of blood
yellow eyes or skin

Spironolactone is an aldosterone agonist, which lowers aldosterone, an adrenal hormone. It works as a diuretic, forcing the dumping of sodium and water. The adrenal glands use sodium to send all their messages to tissues. Aldosterone regulates all body fluids. Spironolactone causes a 100% increase in plasma cortisol levels one hour after administration. The increase in cortisol lasts up to five hours. Given that increased cortisol levels also cause anxiety and an imbalance in the HPA axis, it's clear that given the number of side effects that can occur with spironolactone, taking this drug for acne, which was initially caused by a hormonal imbalance, would further upset the balance.

Common side effects listed by the mayoclinic.org include:[115]

bleeding gums
bloody or black, tarry stools
bloody urine
blurred vision
breast pain
chest pain
clay-colored stools
clear or bloody discharge from the nipple
cloudy urine
confusion
constipation
cough
dark urine
decrease in urine output or decrease in urine-concentrating ability
diarrhea
difficulty with swallowing
dimpling of the breast skin
dizziness
dizziness
drowsiness
fast or irregular heartbeat
fever with or without chills
general feeling of tiredness or weakness
headache
heartburn
hives, itching, or skin rash
hoarseness
increased thirst
indigestion
inverted nipple
loss of appetite

loss of consciousness
lower back or side pain
lump in the breast or under the arm
muscle pain or cramps
muscle spasms or twitching
nausea
painful or difficult urination
persistent crusting or scaling of the nipple
pinpoint red spots on the skin
puffiness or swelling of the eyelids or around the eyes, face, lips, or tongue
redness or swelling of the breast
seizures
severe stomach pain
shakiness and unsteady walk
sore on the skin of the breast that does not heal
sore throat
sores, ulcers, or white spots on the lips or in the mouth
stomach cramping, burning, or tenderness
swelling of the face, fingers, feet, ankles, or lower legs
swollen, painful, or tender lymph glands in the neck, armpit, or groin
tightness in the chest
trembling
troubled breathing
unpleasant breath odor
unsteadiness, trembling, or other problems with muscle control or coordination
unusual bleeding or bruising
unusual tiredness or weakness
vomiting
vomiting of blood or material that looks like coffee grounds
weight gain
yellow eyes or skin
irregular heartbeat
nervousness
numbness or tingling in the hands, feet, or lips
rash with flat lesions or small raised lesions on the skin
reddened skin
weakness or heaviness of the legs
burning feeling in the chest or stomach
decreased interest in sexual intercourse
hair loss or thinning of the hair
inability to have or keep an erection
leg cramps

loss in sexual ability, desire, drive, or performance
pain in the nipples
sores, welts, or blisters
stomach upset
swelling of the breasts or breast soreness in both females and males
unusual dullness or feeling of sluggishness

Eating Disorders

The fasting girls of the 19th century were force-fed, treated with hydrotherapy, institutionalized, and given sedatives. Today, both anorexia nervosa and binge and purging disorders are treated with psychotherapy and antidepressants. I have described the side effects of antidepressants above.

Barrier Method Birth Control

Until the 1960s, the diaphragm was widely used by women for birth control. Although it was promoted in the 1970s as an alternative to hormonal birth control when the women's movement raised concerns about HRT side effects, it is now seldom suggested by gynecologists and certainly not promoted by drug companies. There is less profit in barrier birth control methods. The female condom, which was approved by the FDA in 1993, is largely ignored. Yet health organizations in developing countries promote the female condom because it gives women the right to protect themselves, not only from pregnancy but also from sexually transmitted diseases. The female condom still costs more than the male version because of its lack of popularity, but also because of the pink tax, which means products marketed toward women cost more than those marketed toward men. The fact that it has no side effects and is more protective should make it a more publicized option for women of all ages.

If left to the medical industry and a society whose view of women's health evolved from the 19th century, women will have less control over their bodies. Due to the marketing of the pill, the diaphragm's use plummeted. As of 2014, the most easily used and easily fitting diaphragm, Janssen Pharmaceuticals Inc.'s Ortho-All Flex, was discontinued. Pharmaceutical companies insist that hormonal contraception is more effective than the diaphragm. Drug companies criticize its use because it has to be inserted and removed after eight hours. This means it has to be correctly used to be effective. It is as effective as the male condom. Anything has to be correctly used to be effective.

Women stopped using the diaphragm in the 1980s, and now young women don't even know that this type of barrier to birth control exists as an option. A newer type of barrier method, the Fem-Cap, a cervical cap, is now available in the United States. There are also two other kinds of diaphragms still available in the US. Barrier methods are also a one-time expense, unlike birth control pills. Women have to be fitted for them by a gynecologist, but I think the choice between that inconvenience and dangerous side effects should be an easy one.

The problem with the medications I have described is that their absence is not the cause of the symptoms that occur with each health issue. This is why there are side effects. All medicines have been derived from the plants humans have seen change the degree of symptoms that occur with an illness or disease. A tissue injury will cause a stress response. Our bodies have antiseptic and healing substances that occur naturally. The swelling that comes with a sprained ankle is part of that.

My point is that the medications I list in this chapter are prescribed with the assumption that what is happening in the body is the consequence of a diseased organ when it is not. Female reproductive organs are the same as any other tissue in the body, but medicine, since it evolved from preconceived perceptions of the female body as physiologically inferior, has always treated these organs as prone to disease. They are no more prone to disease than an arm or a foot. The female nervous system has also been traditionally viewed as weaker than the male's, which is why more females are prescribed psychiatric drugs and therapy than males.

But medicine has known since their invention that synthetic estrogens and too much endogenous estrogen cause cervical cancer, breast cancer, and endometrial cancer. When scientists were developing hormone treatments—with massive financing from pharmaceutical companies—few women wanted to be a part of those studies because of the many immediate side effects of vomiting, nausea, dizziness, headaches, and stomach pain. Other side effects included bloating, mood changes, and blood clots, both for menopause and birth control trials. Manufacturers and scientists chose to conduct their trials in low-income Puerto Rican birth control clinics. The doctor in charge of the study of the Enovid clinical trial wrote that it "gives one hundred percent protection against pregnancy [but causes] too many side reactions to be acceptable." Those that could dropped out of the studies.

Americans then tested their pill on women in mental institutions.[116] Schering, the German pharmaceutical giant that is now a part of Bayer, tested their hormone therapies—derived estrogen, progesterone, and testosterone—on Auschwitz prisoners. A recent modern study in 2016 attempted a clinical hormonal birth control study on men, but it was stopped after men reported mood-changing side effects.

Gregory Pincus, who was part of the development team of Enovid, the first FDA-approved synthetic estrogen and progesterone birth control, had tried a hormonal birth control on men. Still, according to Holly Grigg-Spall, in *Sweetening the Pill*, "It was rejected for men due to the number of side effects, including testicle shrinking."[117]

In her *New York Times* article, journalist Katie Rogers argues in favor of hormonal therapy to block menstruation as a means of liberation. As does the advertising campaign for female hormone treatment to treat the brand new illness called "Female Sexual Dysfunction." It includes synthetic estrogen and synthetic testosterone. Women have the right to orgasm, just as they have the right to birth control, but a synthetic hormone with dangerous side effects and surgeries to alter clitoral tissue are not the answer.[118]

Women are led to believe they are ill and that these medical interventions can fix what isn't even broken. Side effects require more medications to silence the negative feedback response to the medication. The idea has long been that if you fix a woman's reproductive system, you've fixed everything that is wrong with her. The discovery of hormones made that bias easier to sell.

The Army Corps of Engineers has been trying to tame the Mississippi River with levees for over 150 years to prevent flooding along its banks. This has only made the flooding worse. Think of medications and the side effects that are part of the negative feedback response as like trying to tame the Mississippi River. Any symptom that signals a health issue is part of the stress response in the body attempting to fix something. Uterine, ovarian, breast tissue fibroids, and cysts are cellular attempts to increase their expanse to trap more iodine from the bloodstream. It is not the shortage of synthetic estrogen and progesterone that has caused the cysts in PCOS, but the inability to properly regulate the secretion of those hormones that occur naturally in ovarian tissue.

There will be a negative feedback response to the exogenous hormones. Why? Because the body did not make them. They are not what the body is asking for. If the ovaries need more iodine and we stick in synthetic hormones, the tissue will have to find another way to signal the need for more iodine, which is usually to grow more cysts. The synthetic hormones will suppress the natural secretion of these hormones, not only in the ovaries but in the adrenals as well. The adrenal glands synthesize 85-90% of the estrogen and progesterone. Since we know estrogen and progesterone receptors are in many tissues, and not only in females, this will have a knock-on effect on the entire endocrine system, which results in side effects.

There are better ways to address the health issues than with medications. We must right the imbalance by providing the missing elements that caused the imbalance in the first place. This is better done naturally and without side effects.

SIX

HOW TO PREVENT AND ADDRESS HEALTH ISSUES DURING PUBERTY AND ADOLESCENCE

I'VE SPENT SEVERAL CHAPTERS DISCUSSING why things can go wrong during a girl's puberty. I have focused on how diet, iodine, and thyroid function affect the smooth transition from a female child's body to a pubertal female's body. In this chapter, I will explain how to prevent and address the symptoms that increasing numbers of girls are experiencing during puberty.

The female body did not evolve to suffer. It is part of the medical male gaze that has associated the female body with a physiological and biological weakness due to a woman's reproductive organs.

The medical biases that our society has created have made females afraid of their bodies. In the past twenty years, I have noticed more men suffering from the same fear that their physiology will suddenly break down. It doesn't work that way. The human body evolved to be resilient and resourceful. Unfortunately, the resourcefulness—the financial gains some professions have reaped from making people afraid of their bodies—has caused this fear.

The only difference between the female and the male body is that females have babies. History has never obsessed so much with the male part of reproduction being inherently dangerous or flawed as it has on the female part. Human males and females evolved to be equal. As I stated, there is only a 5% genetic difference between the male and female bodies. This difference begins to manifest itself at 8 weeks gestation and takes until week 17 to form the differential genitalia for females and males.[1] Prior to this time, the female is indistinguishable from the male fetus.[2] That is where the differences stop. There are no differences in any other organ or tissue in the body.

Males hunted and gathered. Women hunted and gathered. In 1878, the archeologist Hjalmar Stolpe excavated a Viking grave in Birka, Sweden, finding a human skeleton, arrows, shields, a sword, an axe, a spear, and two horses.[3] For 128 years, archeologists assumed the skeleton belonged to a male warrior. "We were blinded by the warrior equipment," said one of the researchers, until they tested DNA from the skeleton and realized they had been wrong.[4] The elite warrior buried with finery was a woman.

The major change in evolution came with agriculture. The advent of agriculture meant the increased consumption of plants and thus the increased consumption of carbohydrates and bread—the supposed staff of life since Mesopotamia. An agricultural society viewed women and their reproductive value as an investment. From an evolutionary perspective, agriculture happened 10,000 years ago or yesterday.[5]

What Happened to Women's Bodies with the Advent of Agriculture?

Paleontologists have demonstrated that osteoporosis, osteoarthritis cavities, and diabetes were first found in skeletal remains from ancient Egypt. The oldest agricultural civilization on record is Mesopotamia. This is when humans first started to use grain as their primary food source. Mesopotamia is considered the heyday of farming communities. While skeletal remains were more difficult to study from Mesopotamia due to the dryer climate and consequent erosion of bone tissue, scientists did note that dental health degenerated with the spread of fructose-rich date palms.[6] The early dynastic Egyptian period came some 1000 years later. It is clear the damage caused by the increased carbohydrate in the human diet was taking its toll by the time paleontologists got their hands on the skeletal remains from this period.

Historically, scientists have viewed the adoption of agriculture as a benefit to humans because it resulted in increased fertility.[7] However, the hypothesis that early menstruation was associated with increased reproductive fitness has been disproven. Increased fertility came at a colossal price. Infant and maternal mortality rates rose precipitously, and human health degenerated worldwide.[8]

By all scientific accounts, human health degenerated with the change from a hunter-gatherer lifestyle to an agricultural one, but for women, it was far worse. Researchers comparing the female pelvic structures of hunter-gatherers and those of agricultural populations found that the hunter-gatherers had much lower rates of perinatal and maternal mortality and that the change in diet created an obstetrical dilemma.

In 1960, S.L. Washburn, trying to explain the obstetrical dilemma of why childbirth is riskier for humans, proposed the hypothesis that as fetal brains became larger and humans stood on two legs, the birth canal became convoluted, and giving birth thus became more problematic.[9] This, he reasoned, was the underlying cause of contemporary fetal and maternal death rates. More recently, paleodemography researchers have been able to conclude that giving birth became dangerous for women when they started to consume predominantly grain instead of hunting and foraging for food.[10]

Hunter-gatherer women were taller than their grain-eating sisters. Lower maternal height is associated with a higher fetal death rate in many populations. Nutritional deficiencies in the mother cause cephalo-pelvic disproportion—when the head of the fetus is bigger than the mother's pelvis and leads to obstructive labor.[11] One of these nutritional deficiencies is Vitamin D.[12] A Vitamin D deficiency is associated with an increased risk of caesarian delivery.[13] Carbohydrate diets cause Vitamin D deficiency. Bone density was 20-30% higher in pre-agricultural humans.[14] The dietary change due to the dependence on agriculture seems to have altered fetal growth patterns. A carbohydrate-rich diet changed the shape of the pelvis and essentially made giving birth more complicated and more dangerous.

With the increased glycemic load in the diet, females menstruated earlier, and maternal and neonatal death rates rose. Hunter-gatherer females had only 3-4 children and had a 3-4 year break between pregnancies. This was because they breastfed their children until they were three to four years of age, and sometimes longer. Nursing suppresses ovulation. Earlier menarche is also associated with a carbohydrate-rich diet. One of the reasons hunter-gatherers females did not start menstruating until 17 or 18 is their high protein and animal fat diet, which was low in carbohydrates. In the 3 to 4 years between pregnancies, mothers could recover nutritionally and ensure they and their offspring were healthy during the pregnancy.

Women in agricultural communities became shorter. The Europeans who migrated to America were much shorter in stature than the ones. They and their progeny started eating abundant meat that poorer European people could not afford. Water sources in agricultural communities were also deficient in minerals. Grain production came from the fact that humans stayed in one place. They stopped being nomadic because they had such a rich source of meat. When that started to run out, they started selecting grass seeds, and grain farming was born. The grain allowed humans to stay in one place, but they became malnourished from eating it. Eating a diet of primary grain gave rise to tooth decay, iron deficiency, cholera, tuberculosis, smallpox, flu, measles, leprosy, syphilis, malaria, the plague, and recurring famine.[15]

The dependence on agriculture created labor divisions between males and females, but it also created class divisions.[16] Hunter-gatherer societies were egalitarian. There was no surplus because a nomadic lifestyle dictated that you only owned what you could carry. All food and materials were shared equally.[17]

Agriculture also brought sexual discrimination. No longer nomadic, women in agricultural societies had more pregnancies.[18] The anthropologist and evolutionary biologist Jared Diamond has written about how women were turned into beasts of burden and carried more than their weight on their backs when men walked empty-handed.[19] Agriculture turned women into breeding machines that existed only to put more people to work in the fields. Female attractiveness and traits of fertility became more important than the female herself. This is the point in history when women became objectified for their looks. This body objectification is the reason why girls are self-conscious about their looks today.

All humans suffer in farming communities, yet women suffer more since women do the same kind of manual labor that males do, even though they traditionally get less meat than males.[20] Adolescent anemia is a massive problem in developing and developed countries.[21] Young females need more iron and need to increase their storage iron to meet future demands of pregnancy.

The reduced consumption of animal foods causes iron deficiency found globally in females. In developing countries, women get less meat to eat. Bushmeat, the primary animal food source in African countries, is consumed by men more than women.[22] In developed countries, low socioeconomic status dictates how much iron females get. Still, females who grow up in prosperous families often refuse to eat meat due to anxiety about gaining weight because of the feminine ideal that evolved in the mid-19th century. Eating meat, or eating at all, is not considered feminine. It is considered masculine.

Even though fertility is hugely expensive, all agricultural societies give women less meat. Agricultural communities in Nepal and India also shun and isolate women in menstruation huts during their cycle. Still, the idea that a woman is impure during menstruation has been an issue in almost all societies since the advent of agriculture. Sir James Frazer, a Scottish anthropologist in the Victorian Era, wrote that societies feared menstrual blood.[23] While this book is not about pregnancy, the scientific explanation of how women's bodies, specifically their menstrual cycles, changed with the advent of agriculture gives us enough proof to demonstrate how diet is crucial to a pubertal female's health.

In developing countries, where men are seen as the heads of the household, men get more meat, and women and children get vegetables and grain. One paper states that gender decides who gets animal-sourced foods in households.[24] The power dynamics and social systems that have evolved since the advent of agriculture decide that women get less meat in the households even though women need it more. Not even addressing the current scientific and medical bias against meat-eating, meat-eating has historically been associated with masculinity. Non-animal-source foods, such as salad, grains, and vegetables, are considered feminine.[25] Men are supposed to get big and strong eating red meat, while women who have 8 to 12 children in agricultural societies and who also have to engage in backbreaking farm work are prevented from eating meat when they most need it. An elderly Italian patient described how her mother used to scrape the pot meat was roasted in, showing me how she pushed the spoon along the inside of the pot with her forearms after giving her husband and sons much larger portions of meat than she gave herself and her daughters.

The result of inadequate animal-source foods for women is higher rates of anemia in women and children globally. This also means higher rates of congenital diseases and illnesses for both women and their children. One paper asks this ridiculous question, "Do biological differences between men and women, such as testosterone levels, have an impact on food preferences?"[26]

The answer is no. Our cultural associations with meat have plagued us since the Victorian era, causing women in prosperous communities to choose not to eat meat. In societies of lower economic status, women do not have the choice to decide to eat meat. They are prevented from eating more meat, even though they want to eat more meat and give their children more meat.

A diet high in meat allowed human parents to care for their offspring into early adulthood. No other primate takes care of its offspring for such an extended amount of time. Humans evolved because they could depend on a rich food resource, which gave us an extended developmental period, intelligence, and a long adult lifespan unique to our species.

Three major components are necessary to prevent health issues in adolescent females—fat, protein, and iodine. How well puberty develops will affect a woman's health for the rest of her life. I look at puberty as the birth of the fertile woman, just as menopause is the birth of the woman who will live up to 50 years as an infertile being who evolved to ensure the well-being of her family and community. This birth requires a diet rich in the essential ingredients that make the endocrine system function optimally. None of these ingredients are found in plants.

Diet

To prevent the health issues associated with puberty, girls need to eat animal protein and animal fat, but specifically red meat as well. The growth spurt triggered by adrenarche demands amino acids and Vitamin D. It has nothing to do with sun exposure. Inuit communities did not have Vitamin D deficiencies until the arrival of carbohydrates brought by Europeans.[27] Animal fat is the supreme source of Vitamin D. The Inuit diet was low in carbohydrates and high in meat and cholesterol. They also breastfed their children longer than Europeans. Today, we don't hear about osteomalacia or rickets as an adolescent illness in the West. Yet, it is associated with puberty in the developed countries of Asia, Southeast Asia, and North Africa.[28]

Most people who have heard of rickets will assume it is a disease of the past. Tiny Tim in Charles Dicken's *A Christmas Story* suffered from rickets because his mother had several children—Tiny Tim was the youngest—and his family was poor. Charles Dickens used his story to bring attention to the malnutrition poor people suffered in nineteenth-century England. Unfortunately, rickets, first described in the 17th century, is back, with rising rates in the industrialized world, including Dickens' England.[29] If we remember that hunter-gatherers had much higher bone density due to their diet high in animal fat, we can understand why there is an increase in rickets.

Adolescents need to eat red meat from ruminant animals, such as beef, lamb, goat, and bison, because it is rich in iron and has the most bioavailable form of all the vitamins and minerals humans evolved to eat. Other forms of animal proteins that are not ruminant, such as fish, poultry, and pork, are rich in amino acids but not as rich in iron. Due to their grain-based diet, chicken and pork have a higher omega-6 content. Seafood does not offer adequate fat. While some people are told they are allergic to iodine and should avoid seafood, there is very little iodine in seafood. One can of sardines provides only 35 mcg of iodine, whereas the growing female body requires so much more. The diet does not have to be only ruminant meat, but it should be the backbone of the diet.

Carbohydrates are not necessary but are what most girls think they should eat. Phytic acid in the hulls of nuts, seeds, and grains prevents the absorption of calcium and other essential nutrients. The problem with plants is the anti-nutrients.[30] Protease inhibitors reduce protein absorption by interfering with pancreatic enzymes, trypsin, and chymotrypsin, breaking down dietary protein. They are found in vegetables such as cereal grains, onions, and peanuts. Oxalates, found in most plant foods, are exceptionally high in green leafy vegetables, soy, almonds, potatoes, tea, rhubarb, cereal grains, and beets. Oxalates reduce iron absorption. Tannins found in legume seeds, cider, cereals, cacao, peas, leafy and green vegetables, coffee, tea, and nuts also reduce iron absorption. Plants in the brassica or cruciferous family are goitrogens. Goitrogens reduce iodine absorption. Thiouracil, one of the first drugs to treat hyperthyroidism, was isolated after a farmer saw that his rabbits developed goiter from eating cabbage leaves. Currently, methimazole, a derivative of the highly toxic thiouracil, is still used to prevent the synthesis of iodine even in iodine-sufficient people. But soy, millet, sweet potatoes, and cassava are also goitrogens. Phytate in grains, beans, nuts, and seeds also reduces iron absorption and the synthesis of zinc, calcium, and magnesium. Beans, which are full of lectins and have become the protein source for those who do not have access to meat, not only disrupt the absorption of iron, calcium, zinc, and magnesium but can also cause gut permeability. Lectins are found in various plant foods, including peanuts, lentils, tomatoes, potatoes, eggplant, fruits, wheat, and other grains.

Plant fiber is indigestible and irritates intestinal tissue, increases gut wall permeability, and leads to diverticulitis, hemorrhoids, intestinal dysbiosis, and constipation. All of the above will lead to inflammation, oxidations, insulin resistance, hormonal dysregulation, and micronutrient deficiencies linked to all non-communicable illnesses, both bodily and mental, preventing healing and causing degeneration.[31]

Humans are brilliant. Cultures with less access to meat, when they became sedentary agricultural communities had to figure out how to make these new foods less poisonous. With trial and error, they figured out that cooking and fermenting plants could neutralize some plant toxins. But to what extent? Countless papers have been written on the benefits of plant compounds, from broccoli's phytochemicals to lectins' supposed antioxidant and anti-inflammatory benefits. They are supposedly full of vitamins and minerals but less so in their cooked form, which is the only way to render beans not poisonous. Furthermore, while they are a cheap alternative to the more bioavailable nutrients in meat and fat, we can look at the invention of folic acid or folate to understand how plants have changed from being the filler in a low-meat diet to the dietary savior of all human health issues, which I have shown were nonexistent until the advent of agriculture.

Biochemist Lucy Wills isolated what was for years called the Wills Factor in 1931 while researching macrocytic anemia and pregnancy among poor Muslim women working in textile factories in Mumbai, India.[32] Even though Muslim Indian families do eat some meat, they are still 67% vegetarian, especially those who are poor. The poor women were given both crude liver extracts and pure liver extracts containing arsenic. Another group of patients received an injection of a liver extract. The women in both groups improved, although a Wikipedia description of Lucy Wills's work states the opposite.[33]

Once she returned to England, she worked at a different hospital, continuing to treat pregnant women with macrocytic anemia. She kept careful records of her patients' diets: bread, fish, white meat, sugary milk, and little vegetables and fruit. Wills herself stated that she considered the liver extract the best treatment for her patients, as opposed to the Marmite or Brewer's yeast, which contained the subsequently named "Wills Factor." Wills own summary of her work when she returned to England stated that she chose the Marmite, or yeast therapy, because it was cheaper.[34]

Synthetic folate was isolated by Herschel K. Mitchell, Esmond E. Snell, and Roger J. Williams in 1941 from 4 lbs of spinach.[35] It became a B vitamin called B 9. The benefit of this folic acid, as it was named, replacing the name of Wills Factor, was that it was cheaper than a meat extract. Previously, no one needed folate. They just ate meat. Today, most blood tests include a test for folic acid. Folic acid is not necessary and is not an essential nutrient. B12 does just fine without it.

I used a high-fat carnivore diet to improve many different health issues in my adult patients. Adolescent patients who have not ingested seed oils and eaten a high carbohydrate diet for decades will not need to remove all plants from their diets as long as they eat a good amount of ruminant meat and fat. When several teenage patients with amenorrhea or painful menstrual cycles added meat to their diets, their symptoms improved after only a couple of months, as long as they were also supplementing with Lugol's iodine.

Iodine

Though the Chinese had been using burnt sponges to treat goiter since 3600 BC, iodine was discovered by accident in the West until 1811. Bernard Courtois noticed a purple vapor rising from a combination of seaweed and sulphuric acid while trying to extract the sodium salts needed to make gunpowder.[36]

The incidence of goiter had only been documented in mountainous areas such as Switzerland and Bolivia. Swiss physicians had to treat a higher incidence of goiter and congenital hypothyroidism, then called cretinism, which caused stunted growth and severe lack of fetal neurodevelopment. J. F. Coindet observed that treating his patients with iodine mixed with distilled alcohol reduced his patients' goiters. Theodore Kocher, another Swiss physician who was renowned for the number of thyroidectomies he performed, discovered that his patients became severely ill when he removed part of the thyroid gland and often died when he removed all of it.[37] French physician Jean Lugol made iodine crystals soluble in water by mixing them with potassium iodide and distilled water in 1829.[38]

The impact of iodine deficiency on adolescent girls wasn't understood until 1917 after David Marine's research involving 2100 adolescent girls demonstrated a considerable decrease in goiter in Ohio, part of the mid-west US goiter belt. Iodized salt went on the market in 1924, and while the small quantity of sodium iodide in the salt did prevent goiter, it did not prevent hypothyroidism.[39] The rate of Hashimoto's thyroiditis, which is named for the presence of lymphocytes and nodular colloid goiter in thyroid tissue, increased dramatically in the US with the consumption of iodized salt.

Iodine is necessary for the thyroid to make thyroid hormones. It is also necessary for breast, uterine, and ovarian tissue—all organs that grow larger during puberty, yet physicians warn their patients against supplementing with it. Iodine is crucial for the healthy development of these tissues. It is also essential to proper immune function, but my focus here is on puberty and the organs that change with the development of sexual characteristics. Every study on goiter states that goiter was more prevalent in females, yet no one ever investigated why. J.H. Means, a prominent thyroidologist in the 40s and 50s at Harvard, wrote that "the thyroid merely traps what it needs and lets the rest go to the kidneys for excretion."[40] In his book, *The Endocrine Function of Iodine*, Salter inserts a diagram by A.W. Elmer from 1938 illustrating the many different tissues that use iodine, along with liver, testicles, and ovaries.[41] Strangely, the diagram leaves out breasts. Means finally concluded that hyperthyroidism was caused by stress.

Another problem is the interchangeable use of iodine. Iodine vaporizes when bound to sodium. The countless papers demonstrating changes to thyroid function using sodium iodide need to be taken with a grain of salt, as 47% of the iodide disappears during cooking.[42, 43] The first Lugol's solution was a 15% solution, now called 5% in the US, to make it seem less potent. Papers describing treatment for hyperthyroid goiter use either Lugol's Solution or potassium iodide almost interchangeably as if they were the same thing. They are not. Potassium iodide or sodium iodide is enough to prevent goiter, but not enough to prevent thyroiditis.

Two researchers, Jan Wolff and Israel Lyon Chaikoff, published a paper in 1948 stating that the success Plummer, Boothby and others had using iodine to put Graves disease into remission was that iodine inhibited the normal organification of iodine into thyroid hormone.[44] The Wolff-Chaikoff effect supposedly inhibits the thyroid gland's use of iodide in rats, rendering them hypothyroid and causing goiters. Despite this claim, the rats did not become hypothyroid. Wolff-Chaikoff never measured the rats' thyroid hormone levels.[45] Even so, the supposed Wolff-Chaikoff effect was assumed to occur in humans. What happened was that the thyroid absorbed the iodine, and on achieving sufficiency, the rats' thyroid glands stopped trapping iodine. Furthermore, Wolff and Chaikoff injected five times the quantity of all the iodine in the rat thyroid with potassium iodide with a radioactive tracer. They were not injected with iodine but radioactive potassium iodide, which creates iodine deficiency.

The medical industry—physicians, associations, and publications accepted this W-C effect as proven and demonized. What was not demonized, yet which did have terrible effects on thyroid function, were radioactive iodine and medications such as methimazole, propylthiouracil, and beta-blocker, which all successfully blocked thyroid activity.[46] Plummer and Boothby used 90 mg of Lugol's solution to normalize thyroid hormone production in a hyperthyroid state without damaging the gland. Wolff claimed any iodine excess to be more than 200 micrograms. That's 5 cans of sardines. They also implied the only organ iodine was essential for was the thyroid gland.

Due to the W-C effect, people fear natural organic iodine supplements, such as Lugol's solution. The fact that women suffer more of both hypo- and hyperthyroidism due to iodine deficiency because they need more iodine than men due to the massive need for iodine and thyroid hormone in adolescence and pregnancy is completely overlooked.

In 1966, Russian scientists gave 200 women suffering from breast pain 10-20 mg of elemental iodine. Their theory was that excess estrogens caused by ovarian cysts due to iodine deficiency had created "dyshormonal hyperphasia of the mammary glands."[47] After 3 months, there was no more breast pain, and the ovarian cysts started to shrink.

How much iodine these tissues need depends on many factors. Testing for iodine levels is very confusing since the official required daily amount of the mineral has been reduced to 150 mcg since Wolff-Chaikoff's problematic paper. Clinicians agree that urine testing is the most accurate, but most doctors only ask for iodine blood levels as this test is cheaper.[48] However, any iodine level test results in a false measurement if substances that block iodine receptors, such as bromide, fluoride, chloride, and perchlorates commonly found in drinking water, are not measured as well. If testing parameters use the 150 mcg cut-off, most people supplementing with Lugol's will be told they have too much iodine in their system. The only accurate test is a 24-hour loading test that Hakala Labs offers.[49] For this test, the measure of iodine sufficiency is if 90% of the 50 mg of iodine ingested before the test is retained after measuring 24 hours' worth of urinary secretion. The 50 mg versus 150 mcg is a vast difference. The 50 mg is 333 times 150 mcg.

For example, large breasts need more iodine. Stress increases the need for iodine and low iodine levels increase stress.[50] Substances that interfere with iodine absorption are not confined to broccoli and cabbage but include fluoride found in many water sources, toothpaste, as well as goitrogenic chemicals put in water bottles, canned foods, and cosmetic products, such as mascara, lipsticks, face and eye makeup and nail polish. If your foundation is smooth and silky, it contains bisphenol-A, an endocrine disruptor, because estrogen receptors can mistake it for estrogen. Bisphenol-A is also a goitrogen. Thus, more iodine may be needed initially to remove these chemicals from the system.[51] A minimum of 4 drops of Lugol's 5% would ensure the thyroid, breast, uterine, and ovarian tissue get all they need for proper functioning and development. The thyroid needs 6 mg. Breast tissue needs 5 mg.[52] If each drop of Lugol's 5% provides 6.25 mg, we are already at 2 drops of Lugol's 5%, and that doesn't leave any for uterine and ovarian tissue. J.H. Means noted that menstruation increased the need for iodine by 15%.[53] In the case of chemical toxicity, there may be a need for a salt-loading protocol to remove the chemicals from the iodine receptors.

Adrenal Function

The adrenals synthesize 85-90% of steroid hormones in the human body. The ovaries synthesize a small amount, but that synthesis is primarily necessary to generate the follicles in the ovaries This follicle production starts with primordial follicles in the female fetus about the 12th week of gestation.[54] Many follicles function as a reservoir for future fertility. After the menarche phase of puberty, with the first menstrual cycle, primordial follicles transition to primary follicles, of which one will become one dominant follicle, producing an egg. If that egg is fertilized, more significant amounts of estrogen and progesterone will be necessary to build the placenta in the endometrium. The adrenal glands are also a source of estrogen before, during, and after pregnancy.[55]

The stress response is made out of cholesterol. While the liver produces a small amount (cholesterol is so essential the body ensures a minimum in circulation), this is not enough to make hormones, regenerate brain tissue, or the myelin sheaths covering the nerves that comprise the central nervous system. This makes it clear why dietary fat is so crucial for health. Unfortunately, endocrinology and medicine have been hung up on the ovarian synthesis of steroid hormones because our culture, since the advent of agriculture that created medicine, explains the entirety of a woman's being through the prism of her reproductive organs.

The fact that the adrenals make most of the steroid hormones necessary for the human body, both male and female, was not discovered until the 1980s by Fernand Labrie.[56] Synthetic hormones are an incredibly lucrative business, and for this reason, the idea that if anything goes wrong in a woman's body (the brain is a part of the body, as are her moods), females are told to fix it with exogenous steroid hormones, despite the proof that they cause harm. Just eat fat. If you eat fat, you will have raw materials for the adrenals to synthesize all the steroid hormones you need from birth to death. If you get pregnant, your ovaries will make some out of fat.

Of course, certain things can interfere with this easy synthesis of hormones from the much-demonized LDL that dietary cholesterol provides. Stress needs a lot of cortisol. The stress response, be it to address arguing with your family, fighting with your friends, worrying about grades, or the inflammation that results from a diet deficient in the nutrients I described above, uses cortisol to mount a defense against not only infection and illness but also the barrage of signals that come from the central nervous system via neurotransmitters—dopamine, serotonin, epinephrine/adrenalin, norepinephrine/noradrenalin—when anything that causes stress occurs. If too much cortisol is needed to address stress, the cholesterol will be used to make cortisol, not the other steroid hormones that make up the rest of the steroid hormones cascade. Estradiol and testosterone are the last hormones synthesized in this cascade of conversions.[57] Their synthesis will not happen smoothly or regularly in long-term stress.

The body does not like extremes. Humans evolved to have the marvelous ability to address stress that keeps our wits about us during danger and allows us to run like hell.

This response can be addictive. People who like jumping out of airplanes, engaging in endurance sports, fighting, staying up late partying or studying, taking saunas, jumping into ice baths, and fasting will seek a stressful lifestyle because the stress response feels so good.[58] It's like any drug. All drugs increase cortisol levels, so they feel good when you are on them. But if you engage in these activities longer than your body can handle, the pituitary gland will turn off the ACTH. This hormone tells the adrenals to secrete cortisol, and you won't make any more cortisol to respond to even small stresses, like not finding your homework or losing your keys. The neurotransmitters running through your nervous system will not stop sending signals to organs that you are under stress (which it perceives as a danger), yet you cannot answer them. Alarms will go off throughout the entire body, but you won't be able to turn them off. This leads to health issues such as asthma, autoimmune conditions, PTSD, depression, and anxiety, as well as the whole array of issues that come from having your steroid hormones synthesized irregularly.[59] You will crave sugar, drugs, and more stress to get that feel-good feeling back.

This brings me to anorexia and self-harm. In the Victorian Era, every single part of a girl's life was under complete control of male authority figures trying to preserve the ideal family structure. Take the family meal as an example. The family meal wasn't as important until the end of the 18th century because most families had an agricultural lifestyle and spent most of their time together throughout the day.

By the middle of the 19th century, eating together as a family had become consecrated as a family reunion since family members were more separated by work and school. Upper and middle-class women were in charge of the family meal. Eating took on more significant importance for mothers to control their children's participation in this ritual and for daughters as a way to wrest themselves free from this control. Sir Horatio Donkin, while agreeing that girls should not be educated because their weak nervous systems would be damaged by the strain, admitted that «the range of activity of women is so limited, and their available paths of work in life so few...that they have not like men, vicarious outlets for feeling in a variety of aims and health pursuits."[60]

In *Fasting Girls*, Joan Blumberg describes how girls who started out starving themselves during the mid-19th-century as a form of agency when subjected to terrible constraints placed on them by society and their parents' attempt to exert moral and physical control over their bodies may have continued to fast because of the raised cortisol levels that occur during fasting that gave them the biochemical equivalent of "runner's high."[61]

"The fact that many anorectics seem unable to eat (or develop withdrawal symptoms when they begin to eat regularly) suggests that something biological as well as psychological is going on."[62]

A form of self-harm, such as cutting, is something I did briefly in the aftermath of terrible fights with the man who would become my first husband. I was 18 at the time, and I remember the sensation of calm I felt after using a kitchen knife to carefully slice into my thigh, somewhere no one would notice. I realize now that I engaged in this form of self-harm as a way to produce the endorphins that would make me feel better after the fights. Any incision on the skin will trigger a surge of cortisol secretion.[63]

Endorphins are what produce the "runner's high." They are opioid peptides produced in a parallel secretion with ACTH by the pituitary gland as part of the stress response. ACTH triggers a release of cortisol from the adrenal glands. The plasma levels of both cortisol and endorphins rise significantly and simultaneously with both physiological and physical stress.

Endorphins, specifically beta-endorphins, are part of the endogenous opioid system.[64] They are as powerful a painkiller as heroin. They also have an anti-inflammatory effect on the brain. Exercise increases endorphin levels, hence the term "runner's high."[65] But so does stress, as they are part of the biochemical response to acute stressors, as is cortisol. However, chronic stress tends to inhibit the release of endorphins. Acute stress triggers a release of both cortisol and beta-endorphins. However, chronic stress will eventually cause a deficiency in both cortisol and beta-endorphins as part of the negative feedback mechanism.[66] Chronic stress leads to low cortisol and endorphin deficiencies because high cortisol levels are inflammatory. Beta-endorphins actually inhibit the immune system's response to stress. The pituitary will eventually downregulate and suspend the secretion of both. This means engaging in behavior that produces these feel-good chemicals will create a deficiency in the stress response. This is what causes depression, PTSD, and asthma.[67, 68]

What To Do?

I've demonstrated how endocrine imbalances can cause the health issues associated with puberty and adolescence. These imbalances are caused by nutritional deficiencies and stress that will disrupt normal endocrine function and also cause anxiety, depression, and inflammation.

Animal fat in the form of cholesterol helps humans address stress. The easiest thing to do is to eliminate the foods and substances that prevent the proper absorption and assimilation of nutrients crucial for a healthy endocrine function, but also ensure that you are not overexerting yourself and relying on stimulants for energy. You will have to inspect what you eat, do, and put on your body and slowly remove everything, preventing your endocrine and stress systems from functioning optimally. That means eating animal fat and reducing or removing carbohydrates because they increase cortisol levels. Synthetic hormones, such as birth control, increase cortisol levels. Make-up that has inflammatory ingredients raises cortisol levels. Over-exercising raises cortisol levels. Cortisol is part of the stress response. If we overuse this stress response, we are abusing it. That is why most of my patients realize their health issues started with puberty.

Society wants us to add things to our diet in the form of supplements and substances we put on our skin. But all supplementation has been developed to add nutrients that are missing from the food we eat. This means buying them from purveyors who will make a profit from you. Young girls using anti-aging creams when they are teenagers is another way to make girls conform to the pursuit of an idea of perfection created during the 19th century.[69] Of course, you want beautiful skin, but a healthy diet that ensures a balanced endocrine system (since androgen hormones are always blamed for acne) is what makes beautiful skin.

Retinol products have been marketed to teens for decades as a treatment for acne and skin blemishes, but if one of the side effects is hypothyroidism, along with the others I listed in Chapter 5, it doesn't make sense to use them. Retinoic acid also raises cortisol synthesis.[70] Imagine the double whammy to your endocrine system—thyroid and cortisol function—these products are.

Human skin thrives on a high-fat carnivore diet. The cholesterol in animal fat makes unblemished and wrinkle-free skin and skin cells elastic and resistant. Skin stuffed with vegetable oils—mono or polyunsaturated, trans fat, becomes damaged. Breasts become fuller on a diet high in animal fat.[71] A Japanese study found that dietary fat reduced skin aging in Japanese women.[72] Why would anyone then need retinol creams?

Plenty of foods, besides sugars, are stimulants and raise cortisol levels, such as the spices cinnamon, cardamom, vanilla, and nutmeg. That pumpkin spice latte that's so popular raises cortisol. Mint and chamomile raise cortisol levels. These spices and herbs are probably the least likely to cause problems unless you have issues with anxiety, concentration, or depression. Yet, it is something to consider. I've had so many patients realize that a particular food they ate all their lives was the culprit of their depression and anxiety. Many of the supplements and foods sold to comfort us are harmful. Plants contain potent chemicals that can be toxic. Vanilla is an opiate.[73]

The fact that it has been used as an antidepressant. A study on mice concluded that 100 mg/kg of vanillin had the same effect as fluoxetine on the mice stressed for the study. The fact that it has been used for its ability to lower anxiety and depression since the 17th century only means that it has the same potent side effects as fluoxetine or any other psychiatric drug. All drugs started as plant chemicals.

Perhaps a small amount used for flavoring is not harmful if nothing else in your system provokes a stress response, but consider the fact that if life is stressful, adding stressful substances to the mix, so you don't feel the stress will cause harm over time, just as a cortisone shot can keep an athlete in the game, but repeated cortisone shots will damage bone, ligament, and muscle tissue, shortening the athlete's career.

Fat lowers cortisol.[74,75] Patients have told me they have addressed panic attacks and pain by eating spoonfuls of butter. If a girl regularly avoids fat, she will not have the cortisol reserve to address stressful life events. Puberty should not be stressful physiologically, but any deficiency in nutrients or iodine will cause stress to the system. Hormones will not be synthesized appropriately during the thyroidarche, adrenarche, pubarche, and menarche stages of puberty. This will lead to the health issues addressed in Chapter 2.

Thyroid Function

The thyroid gland needs 6 milligrams of iodine daily to produce adequate quantities of thyroid hormone and a constant supply of various nutrients from iron to magnesium to Vitamin D.[76] I've explained how these are more bioavailable in animal foods. Iron stores will be low if a girl does not eat red meat. Ruminant meat is richer in vitamins and minerals than other animal protein sources, but all animal protein sources are healthy.

Only dairy can cause problems for the thyroid gland if there is any inflammation due to deficiencies or stress. Dairy milk proteins can be mistaken for viral pathogens by an immune system that turns autoimmune into a stress state.[77] Milk and dairy products contain potent opioids that can turn into exorphins that mimic the feel-good effects of endorphins simply by causing inflammation.[78] Two tablespoons of cow milk have enough casein to hit the digestive system and produce an opioid response.[79] No wonder it is hard for people to give up milk and cheese.

Gluten causes an even more powerful opiate response. Both the opioid-producing peptides in casein and gluten proteins were 10 times stronger than morphine in the brains of rats. Naltrexone, an opioid antagonist used to treat heroin dependence, has been seen to prevent binge eating in humans.[80] The symptoms of patients with mental disturbances such as schizophrenia, bipolar disorder, depression, anxiety, and autism improved on a gluten and casein-free diet. One study demonstrated that depression in women improved when the milk they were drinking was replaced by A2 milk, which has a different casein protein that may be less inflammatory than the casein in A1 milk, the type of milk most dairy cows make.[81] Both sheep and goat milk and some breeds of cows, such as the Jersey and Guernsey cows in some parts of the United Kingdom, produce A2 milk. However, it's best to remove all dairy initially to be certain, and then reintroduce first A2 milk products and then try A1 milk products. In any case, no dairy is necessary for nutrition. Raw dairy has no less lactose or milk protein, so pasteurized or raw doesn't make a difference. Since it's the milk proteins in dairy that can be inflammatory, butter isn't usually a problem.

Young people know about lactose intolerance. For this reason, many drink seed and grain milk, but oat, almond, and soy milk contain lectins and goitrogens. Other alternative kinds of milk, such as coconut and rice, have very low iodine levels. Many countries traditionally have fortified dairy cows with iodine during winter months. Dairy is one of the few sources of iodine in the UK.[82] Milk has been fortified with iodine.

A 2022 Italian paper remarked that infants drinking soy-based formula were likely in danger of developing hypothyroidism and that their diet should be supplemented with iodine.[83] Iodine has been added to most soy-based infant formulas since 1961.[84] Still, physicians in the past have wondered how well the manufacturers removed the goitrogenic substances, such as phyto-estrogenic isoflavonoids, that interfere with the synthesis of thyroid hormone from the soybeans processed for formula.

While cow milk allergies may be one reason many women are avoiding cow milk, the fact that women are told to avoid cholesterol, which plant-based milk is devoid of, is another reason young girls may be avoiding cow milk. In 2022, UK nutrition professor Ian Givens created a stir when he stated in an interview with the *UK Times* that women between the ages of 11 and 18 were deficient in iodine because they ate so little meat and drank more plant-based milk than cow milk.[85]

We are the only mammals that drink another animal's milk. We haven't evolved to eat dairy, which is why so many humans react to it. Humans only started drinking it after the dependence on agriculture led to recurring famine.[86] I don't think taking lactaid because your body is telling you to avoid dairy is an ideal solution. There is also the issue of inflammation caused by dairy proteins. If you don't react to it, a small amount regularly is not harmful, but it's worth a try to see if you feel better removing it. Because it is a wheat protein, gluten is also inflammatory.

A diet with adequate levels of nutrients found in meat and animal fat, as well as the inclusion of two to four drops of Lugol's iodine solution, will ensure a young girl has optimum thyroid function during puberty. There are cases where undiagnosed hypothyroidism can be a problem, requiring more thyroid support, but I have found this in only rare cases of people under 20 years old. A woman who has been hypothyroid during her pregnancy will have to use the fetus' thyroid hormone, which starts being produced at 16 weeks. Overt hypothyroidism will usually be diagnosed at birth, but low thyroid function will often not be clinically investigated in newborns. Doctors are looking for severe signs of hypothyroidism, such as swelling around the eyes. Often, low thyroid function won't manifest until puberty, when no one is looking for it, for all of the reasons I describe in this book, namely the supposed perils of puberty.

Fat Avoidance

Many 19th-century physicians lamented the use of corsets to exaggerate the curves associated with femininity and the avoidance of meat. Victorian middle-class and American Gilded Age females were trying to avoid anything that could be associated with the baser human instincts of sexuality. Lower classes were happy to get as much meat as possible, as meat and milk were often outside their budget. Farm girls were considered robust and not as beautiful as the willowy pale girls of the upper classes. They had access to meat and milk from the animal husbandry still practiced by the farming communities. Factory workers had little access to protein, but these were the girls society was worried about. This fear of the sudden independence groups of females living in cities, far from their families, triggered the massive dichotomy between adolescent females and males in the upper classes.

George Stanley Hall, called "The Male Chauvinist Educator" by Professor Gill Schofer, wrote that boys, to become strong men, had to live a "boy's boy" to become a "man's man."[87] Boyhood activities included "tribal, predatory, hunting, fishing, fighting, roving, idle, playing proclivities," that were normal to boyish "savagery." Hall wrote that girls had to stay home and learn to cook, clean, and sew.[88] His views were a product of the 50 years of physicians, educators, and ministers wringing their hands with worry about the abandonment the factory girl would bring upon the upper and middle-class society. The evangelical movements that influenced culture in the 19th century convinced girls that eating meat and animal fat was unseemly for a docile, asexual girl, which was the ideal of that period.

Mental Health and Hormones

There is a truth to the concern about girls and puberty that began in the mid-19th century. Girls need optimum nutrition because of the increased need for thyroid hormone and iodine beginning with puberty. There is a whole category of research today born from the medical concerns over pubertal girls in the Victorian Era investigating to determine if pubertal girls are more susceptible to mental health issues due to the changes in hormone levels.

Women have historically sought help for depression more than men. The known bias against women in the medical field caused researchers to focus their research on figuring out if women had more mental health issues than men or if this was a result of the historical treatment bias. A large epidemiological study carried out in 1984 by the National Institute of Mental Health found an 8% to 9% higher rate of depression in women than men.[89] Studies focused on the changes in the HPA axis during the menstrual cycle's luteal phase when estrogen and progesterone become lower before rising again.[90] Researchers doubled down to investigate if the prevalence of depression in women could be correlated with changes in levels of sex steroid hormones that are regulated by the HPA axis. These studies would try to eliminate the possibility of bias.

Levels of progesterone and estrogen were measured in depressed women and women who were not depressed. Both depressed and not depressed women had the same levels of progesterone and estrogen. Furthermore, despite the practice of prescribing both hormones to women to improve symptoms of PMS without adequate evidence, researchers found no improvement. D.R. Rubinow concluded that changes in ovarian steroids did not cause PMS but "entrained" to them, meaning it was connected to changing levels but not caused by them.[91] The single isolating factor in common with depression was the HPA axis response to stress through the secretion of cortisol.[92] It was stress, not changes in estrogen or progesterone, that provoked a cortisol response during this period, causing women with PMS to have affective symptoms, such as anxiety, irritability, sadness, lethargy, difficulty concentrating, and aches and pains associated with this part of the menstrual cycle, which starts at day 15 and ends typically at day 28.

Practical Solutions

I recommend 2 drops of 5% Lugol's Iodine Solution for girls starting at 9. There is too much variation for me to recommend a diet, but as long as 4 oz or 100 g of ruminant meat, such as beef and lamb, is eaten daily, the daily requirement of 3 mg of iron will be easily achieved. Other than beef liver, no other protein has that amount of iron. While spinach has the same amount of iron per gram as beef, it is non-heme iron (as the iron in all plants), which the human body does not absorb. About 95% of the functional iron in human tissue is heme iron. Non-heme iron is not an essential nutrient. Heme iron, which only occurs in animal flesh, is an essential nutrient.[93]

Low cholesterol is associated with depression, suicidal ideation, and aggression.[94] The inability to metabolize cholesterol causes inflammation and cell death in tissues. The adrenals are the glands that take up the most cholesterol in the human body. In mice, the adrenals take up 19% of the cholesterol versus 2% in ovarian and testicular tissue.[95] Dietary fat provides the cholesterol necessary to replenish the cortisol needed to address stress, but it is also the only nutrient that lowers the cortisol produced in response to stress. Eating abundant fat will address any physiological inflammatory state and any stress state. How much is needed will vary from person to person. It is enough to say that avoiding animal fat is dangerous.

In every paper I studied in which researchers attempted to correlate a high-fat diet with increased physiological stress, the high-fat food was a combination of trans fat and sugar, such as in a donut.[96] None of these papers tested the effects of animal fat on the stress response. When the effects of dietary fat derived from animal fat are studied, the results are entirely different. In a different study, the cortisol levels of elite runners were studied for two weeks on a high-fat and low-fat diet. The runners on the high-fat diet had lower cortisol levels after training, which means the stress induced by endurance running did not increase inflammation.[97]

Low-fat diets are associated with higher stress, violence, and suicide. One study concluded that a large amount of glucose one hour before a psychosocial stressor increased the cortisol response more than fat and protein. The glucose intensified the stress response, whereas the fat and protein stabilized it. Another study compared the effects of a high-carbohydrate and a high-fat diet.[98] They demonstrated that the high-carbohydrate diet raised levels of anger and hostility, and the high-fat diet lowered anxiety and tension.

It all has to do with serotonin. Stress increases cortisol, and cortisol desensitizes serotonin receptors. Carbohydrates desensitized serotonin receptors, but dietary fat did not. Omega-3 fatty acids improve serotonin levels and have the same effect on stabilizing mood as potent mood stabilizers. Only animal fat has omega-3 fatty acids. It doesn't have to come from fish. Butter and beef fat have plenty. Since cholesterol has been demonized, Omega-6 fatty acids from nuts and seed oils have increased in our diet. High Omega-6 levels are associated with depression, alcoholism, and mental disturbances due to their inflammatory nature.[99]

I recommend girls eat fatty meat and supplement with Lugol's 5% iodine. The fatty meat and iodine will provide all the necessary nutrients and fat to ensure the endocrine system is balanced. Both my daughters follow this plan. Once all symptoms have improved, you can consider eating the occasional carbohydrate and dairy, but remember, these are not necessary for nutrition. They will always be entertainment. It is easy to remove them if stress increases. I rarely do, but I eat this way so I can go paddleboarding as much as I can and to make sure I never get the Alzheimer's Disease my mother had. There are plenty of resources if you are curious about the carnivore diet. I recommend Judy Cho's new book, *The Complete Carnivore Diet for Beginners: Your Practical Guide to an All-Meat Lifestyle.* It will have the answers to any questions you might have. It's pretty simple, though. You eat all animal foods and ensure you eat extra fat if you eat chicken and fish. It's always important to eat red meat so you get enough iron. Add salt and water, and you have a perfect diet. If that sounds boring, remember that most people eat the same foods every day because they like them. This is eating the same foods every day because you feel good. And you don't have to eat the same foods every day. There are many different kinds of animal foods to choose from. This is how humans evolved to eat.

I spent two years wanting to be a boy. From eight to ten, I thought only boys would have fun. I wore my long blonde hair in a ponytail and stared at myself in the mirror, trying to see the boy I would be, who was called Jim. I wasn't interested in dolls until my mother (despite her feminist concerns about Barbies) gave me a Barbie for Christmas when I was ten. I promptly constructed bathroom sinks out of seashells for her. I wasn't that interested in her outfits. When my mother bought me a Ken doll, I had him and Barbie do what I thought my mother and her friends did with their boyfriends.

My two older children's experiences with psychiatrists and rehabilitation centers illustrate how differently a teenage girl and a teenage boy are treated by medicine. They have three near overdoses between them. My daughter became bulimic after taking the pill for contraception at 15. She took it against my advice and immediately gained weight. She also started drinking heavily, enough for the police in our small town in Italy to regularly bring her to the emergency room. My son started experimenting with drugs during college.

These memories are harrowing, but if I fast-forward several years to them both being in drug rehab centers in the same area of Italy where we lived, I see how different my daughter's treatment was from my son's. My daughter was diagnosed with borderline personality. She was given a chemical straitjacket of mood stabilizers and antidepressants. She lived in a building in the hills with many other young women and a smattering of males. She had regular psychiatric evaluations. She had no activities, save for trips into town with me and my husband so she could have coffee.

My son was not given any diagnosis at all. He was not put on any medication but offered a weekly therapy session. He was given an opportunity to learn different skills, a room to teach other young men how to play an instrument, and access to a weight room. My son spent two years and a half years there. He left six months early because his father was ill with cancer. He has rebuilt his life and is now thriving.

My daughter spent ten years in and out of different psychiatric wards and a total of 6 years in one particular rehab community. Her rights were taken away from her by a judge, and she became a ward of the Italian state. I finally put her on a plane to Greece, where her brother lives. She started the long process of weaning off of the chemicals. Even though she lost ten years of her life to the chemical straitjacket and a diagnosis I never agreed with, she is now starting a new career at 35 and also thriving.

This personal story explains why this book is so important to me. I hope that reading about how our definition of what a girl should do and be was created by a society that had no interest in the health of girls or women will help girls understand and question their assumptions and even what medicine tells them is the way to live a happy and healthy life. Puberty and being female have been medicalized for too long. If we can eat in a way that gives us the essential nutrients for our endocrine system to find balance, limit toxins, and not create a further imbalance by adding pharmaceuticals, we can help young girls grow into happy and healthy women.

ENDNOTES

ONE
THE PERILS OF PUBERTY

1 https://www.theatlantic.com/newsletters/archive/2022/04/american-teens-sadness-depression-anxiety/629524/. Accessed December 19, 2023.

2 https://www.economist.com/united-states/2017/11/23/teenagers-are-growing-more-anxious-and-depressed.

3 https://www.nytimes.com/2023/03/23/opinion/cdc-teenagers.html?smid=url-share. Accessed December 19, 2023.

4 https://www.nytimes.com/2023/03/23/opinion/cdc-teenagers.html

5 https://www.nytimes.com/2023/05/23/health/surgeon-general-social-media-mental-health.html?smid=nytcore-ios-share&referringSource=articleShare. Accessed December 19, 2023.

6 https://www.nytimes.com/2023/02/13/health/teen-girls-sadness-suicide-violence.html?smid=nytcore-ios-share&referringSource=articleShare. Accessed December 19, 2023.

7 Naz MSG, Tehrani FR, Majd HA, Ahmadi F, Ozgoli G, Fakari FR, Ghasemi V. "The Prevalence of Polycystic Ovary Syndrome in Adolescents: A Systematic Review and Meta-Analysis. *Int J Reprod Biomed.* 2019 Sep 3;17(8):533-542.

8 Andrea D. Coviello, Richard S. Legro, Andrea Dunaif. "Adolescent Girls with Polycystic Ovary Syndrome Have an Increased Risk of the Metabolic Syndrome Associated with Increasing Androgen Levels Independent of Obesity and Insulin Resistance." *The Journal of Clinical Endocrinology & Metabolism*, Volume 91, Issue 2, 1 February 2006, Pages 492–497.

9 Sieberg C B, Lunde CE, Boorsook D. "Endometriosis and Pain in the Adolescent--Striking Early to Limit Suffering: A Narrative Review." Neuroscience & Biobehavioral Reviews Volume 108,2020, Pages 866-876

10 Hirsch M, Dhillon-Smith R, Cutner AS, Yap M, Creighton SM. "The Prevalence of Endometriosis in Adolescents with Pelvic Pain: A Systematic Review." *J Pediatr Adolesc Gynecol.* 2020 Dec;33(6):623-630.

11 Wilson S, Dumornay NM. "Rising Rates of Adolescent Depression in the United States: Challenges and Opportunities in the 2020s." *J Adolesc Health.* 2022 Mar;70(3):354-355.

12 https://www.pewresearch.org/short-reads/2019/07/12/a-growing-number-of-american-teenagers-particularly-girls-are-facing-depression/. Accessed December 19, 2023.

13 Angold, A., Costello, E., and Worthman, C. (1998). "Puberty and Depression: The Roles of Age, Pubertal Status and Pubertal Timing." *Psychological Medicine, 28*(1), 51-61.

14 Hochberg ZE, Konner M. "Emerging Adulthood, a Pre-adult Life-History Stage." *Front Endocrinol* (Lausanne). 2020 Jan 14;10:918.

15 Hall, G. S. (1904). *Adolescence: Its Psychology and Its Relations to Physiology, Anthropology, Sociology, Sex, Crime, Religion and Education*, Vol. 1. D Appleton & Company.

16 Dubas, Judith Semon et al. "The Study of Adolescence during the 20th Century." *The History of the Family* 8 (2003): 375 - 397.

17 Arnett JJ. "Emerging Adulthood: A Theory of Development from the Late Teens through the Twenties." *Am Psychol.* (2000) 55:469. 10.1037/0003-066X.55.5.469

18 Arain M, Haque M, Johal L, Mathur P, Nel W, Rais A, Sandhu R, Sharma S. "Maturation of the Adolescent Brain." *Neuropsychiatr Dis Treat.* 2013;9:449-61

19 Hochberg, Z. (2012). *Evo Devo of Child Growth: Treatize on Child Growth and Human Evolution.* New York, NY: Wiley.

20 Hochberg Z, Gawlik A, Walker RS. "Evolutionary Fitness as a Function of Pubertal Age in 22 Subsistence-Based Traditional Societies." *Int J Pediatr Endocrinol.* 2011;2011(1):2.

21 Shostak, Marjorie. Nisa: *The Life and Words of a !Kung Woman.* Harvard University Press, 1981

22 Gluckman PD & Hanson MA. "Evolution, Development and Timing of Puberty." *Trends in Endocrinology and Metabolism* 2006 17 7–12.

23 https://www.nytimes.com/2012/04/01/magazine/puberty-before-age-10-a-new-normal.html

24 Belsky J, Steinberg L, Houts RM, Halpern-Felsher BL, NICHD Early Child Care Research Network. "The Development of Reproductive

Strategy in Females: Early Maternal Harshness –> Earlier Menarche –> Increased Sexual Risk Taking." *Dev Psychol.* (2010) 46:120–8.

25 Euling SY, Selevan SG, Pescovitz OH, Skakkebaek NE. "Role of Environmental Factors in the Timing of Puberty." *Pediatrics.* 2008 Feb;121 Suppl 3:S167-71.

26 Jean Claude Carel, Najiba Lahlou, Marc Roger, Jean Louis Chaussain. "Precocious Puberty and Statural Growth." Human Reproduction Update, Volume 10, Issue 2, March 2004, Pages 135–147

27 Mendle J, Moore SR, Briley DA, Harden KP. "Puberty, Socioeconomic Status, and Depression in Girls: Evidence for Gene × Environment Interactions." *Clin Psychol Sci.* 2016 Jan 1;4(1):3-16

28 Graber JA. "Pubertal Timing and the Development of Psychopathology in Adolescence and Beyond." *Horm Behav.* 2013 Jul;64(2):262-9

29 https://time.com/6255448/teen-girls-mental-health-epidemic-causes/

30 Skovlund CW, Kessing LV, Mørch LS, Lidegaard Ø. "Increase in Depression Diagnoses and Prescribed Antidepressants among Young Girls." A national cohort study 2000-2013. *Nord J Psychiatry.* 2017 Jul;71(5):378-385.

31 https://www.cdc.gov/nchs/products/databriefs/db283.htm#:~:text=Females were approximately twice as, medication at all time points.

32 Hochberg, Z. (2012). *Evo Devo of Child Growth: Treatize on Child Growth and Human Evolution.* New York, NY: Wiley.

33 Ibid.

34 Gluckman PD & Hanson MA. "Evolution, Development and Timing of Puberty." *Trends in Endocrinology and Metabolism* 2006 17 7–12.

35 Mendle J, Moore SR, Briley DA, Harden KP. "Puberty, Socioeconomic Status, and Depression in Girls: Evidence for Gene × Environment Interactions." *Clin Psychol Sci.* 2016 Jan 1;4(1):3-16

36 Steinberg L. "A Social Neuroscience Perspective on Adolescent Risk-Taking." *Dev Rev.* 2008 Mar;28(1):78-106.

37 Collado-Rodriguez A, MacPherson L, Kurdziel G, Rosenberg LA, Lejuez CW. "The Relationship between Puberty and Risk Taking in the Real World and in the Laboratory." *Pers Individ Dif.* 2014 Oct 1;68:143-148.

38 Ibid.

39 Lerner, R. M., & Steinberg, L. (2009). "The Scientific Study of Adolescent Development: Historical and Contemporary Perspectives." In R. M. Lerner & L. Steinberg (Eds.), *Handbook of Adolescent Psychology:*

Individual Bases of Adolescent Development (pp. 3–14). John Wiley & Sons, Inc..

40 Buchanan C, Eccles J, Becker J. "Are Adolescents the Victims of Raging Hormones? Evidence for Activational Effects of Hormones on Moods and Behavior at Adolescence." *Psychological Bulletin.* 1992;111:62–107

41 Hall, G. S. (1904). *Adolescence: Its Psychology and Its Relations to Physiology, Anthropology, Sociology, Sex, Crime, Religion and Education*, Vol. 1. D Appleton & Company.

42 G. Stanley Hall to Sigmund Freud, letter of 15 December 1908, reprinted in S. Rosenzweig, *The Historic Expedition to America (1909): Freud, Jung and Hall the King-Maker* (St. Louis: Rana House, 1994), p. 339.

43 Demos, John, and Virginia Demos. "Adolescence in Historical Perspective." *Journal of Marriage and Family*, vol. 31, no. 4, 1969, pp. 632–38. *JSTOR*, https://doi.org/10.2307/349302. Accessed 10 Dec. 2023.

44 Loke KY, Viner RM. "The Perils of Puberty." *Ann Acad Med Singap.* 2003 Jan;32(1):3-6.

45 Parameswaran, G. (2020). The social historical roots of the concept of emerging adulthood and its impact on early adults. *Theory & Psychology, 30*(1), 18-35.

46 *A Doctor of Their Own: The History of Adolescent Medicine*. By Heather Munro Prescott (Cambridge: Harvard University Press, 1998. xi plus 238pp.

47 Ibid.

48 Smith BH & Tompkins RL. "Toward a Life History of the Hominidae." *Annual Review of Anthropology* 1995 24 257–279.

49 *A Doctor of Their Own: The History of Adolescent Medicine*. By Heather Munro Prescott (Cambridge: Harvard University Press, 1998. xi plus 238pp.

50 Ibid

51 *Handbook of Adolescent Psychology*, New Jersey: Wiley & Sons , 1980

52 Hall, G. S. (1904). *Adolescence: Its Psychology and Its Relations to Physiology, Anthropology, Sociology, Sex, Crime, Religion and Education*, Vol. 1. D Appleton & Company.

53 Weeks, J. (2017). *Sex, Politics and Society: The Regulation of Sexuality Since 1800* (4th ed.). Routledge.

54 https://www.haaretz.com/archaeology/2023-04-10/ty-article/the-rules-of-masturbation-in-ancient-greece/00000187-6a8d-d484-adef-ea8de62d0000. Accessed December 19, 2023.

55 Marland, Hilary Unstable Adolescence: "Medicine and the 'Perils of Puberty' in Late Victorian and Edwardian Britain, Health and Girlhood in Britain, 1874-1920." *Palgrave Studies in the History of Childhod*, pg 15-41

56 Weeks, J. (2017). *Sex, Politics and Society: The Regulation of Sexuality Since 1800* (4th ed.). Routledge.

57 "The Brutal Anti-Masturbation Devices of the Victorian Era." news.com.au, By LJ Charleston 20 Jul, 2019 10:53 PM, accessed December 10, 2023

58 Marland, H. "Unstable Adolescence: Medicine and the 'Perils of Puberty' in Late Victorian and Edwardian Britain, Health and Girlhood in Britain, 1874-1920." *Palgrave Studies in the History of Childhood*, pg 15-41

59 Ibid.

60 Brumberg J J. *The Body Project: An Intimate History of American Girls.* New York: Random House, 1997.

61 Op de Macks ZA, Bunge SA, Bell ON, Wilbrecht L, Kriegsfeld LJ, Kayser AS, Dahl RE. "Risky Decision-Making in Adolescent Girls: The Role of Pubertal Hormones and Reward Circuitry." *Psychoneuroendocrinology*. 2016 Dec;74:77-91.

62 Hur JH, Park S, Jung MK, Kang SJ, Kwon A, Chae HW, Kim HS, Kim DH. "Insulin Resistance and Bone Age Advancement in Girls with Central Precocious Puberty." *Ann Pediatr Endocrinol Metab*. 2017 Sep;22(3):176-182

63 Smith, B. Holly, and Robert L. Tompkins. "Toward a Life History of the Hominidae." *Annual Review of Anthropology* 24 (1995): 257–79. http://www.jstor.org/stable/2155938.

64 Gómez-Robles A, Nicolaou C, Smaers JB, Sherwood CC. The evolution of human altriciality and brain development in comparative context. Nat Ecol Evol. 2024 Jan;8(1):133-146.

TWO
A HISTORY OF THE HEALTH ISSUES OF PUBERTAL AND ADOLESCENT GIRLS

1 Weeks, J. (2017). *Sex, Politics and Society: The Regulation of Sexuality Since 1800* (4th ed.). Routledge.

2 Marland, H. (2013). "Unstable Adolescence: Medicine and the 'Perils of Puberty' in Late Victorian and Edwardian Britain." In: *Health and Girlhood in Britain, 1874–1920. Palgrave Studies in the History of Childhood.* Palgrave Macmillan, London

3 Philippe. *Centuries of Childhood; A Social History of Family Life.* New York :Knopf, 1962.

4 Weeks, J. (2017). *Sex, Politics and Society: The Regulation of Sexuality Since 1800* (4th ed.). Routledge, p 61.

5 Voss, B. L. 2006. "Engendered Archaeology: Men, Women, and Others." In *Historical Archaeology*, edited by M. Hall and S. Silliman, pp. 107-127. Blackwell Publishing, London.

6 Laquer, T. *Making Sex: Body and Gender from the Greeks To Freud.* Cambridge: Harvard University Press, 1990.

7 Le Guin, Ursula K. 2018. *The Left Hand of Darkness.* S.F. Masterworks. London, England: Gollancz.

8 Woolf, Virginia. 1995. *Orlando.* Wordsworth Classics. Ware, England: Wordsworth Editions.

9 Laquer, T. *Making Sex: Body and Gender from the Greeks To Freud.* Cambridge: Harvard University Press, 1990.

10 Institute of Medicine (US) Committee on Understanding the Biology of Sex and Gender Differences; Wizemann TM, Pardue ML, editors. *Exploring the Biological Contributions to Human Health: Does Sex Matter?* Washington (DC): National Academies Press (US); 2001.

11 James Gregory. *Of Victorians and Vegetarians: The Vegetarian Movement in Nineteenth-Century Britain.* London: Tauris Academic Studies, 2007

12 Ibid.

13 http://ap.gilderlehrman.org/history-by-era/first-age-reform/essays/sylvester-graham-and-antebellum-diet-reform. Accessed December 18, 2023.

14 Shprintzen, A D. *The Vegetarian Crusade: The Rise of an American Reform Movement, 1817-1921.* University of North Carolina Press, 2013.

15 https://www.theatlantic.com/health/archive/2014/01/looking-to-quell-sexual-urges-consider-the-graham-cracker/282769/. December 18. 2023.

16 https://www.thedailymeal.com/1157662/the-strange-story-behind-the-invention-of-the-graham-cracker/. December 18. 2023.

17 Banta, Jim E., Jerry W. Lee, Georgia Hodgkin, Zane Yi, Andrea Fanica, and Joan Sabate. 2018. "The Global Influence of the Seventh-Day Adventist Church on Diet." *Religions* 9, no. 9: 251.

18 Numbers, R L. Prophetess of Health: A Study of Ellen G. White. New York: Harper & Row, 1976

19 https://www.nonsda.org/egw/contra6.shtml. Accessed December 18, 2023.

20 https://en.wikipedia.org/wiki/John_Harvey_Kellogg. Accessed December 19. 2023.

21 https://www.adventistreview.org/archives/2005-1538/story2.html. December 18. 2023

22 https://en.wikipedia.org/wiki/John_Harvey_Kellogg. Accessed December 19. 2023.

23 Money J. *The Destroying Angel : Sex, Fitness & Food in the Legacy of Degeneracy Theory : Graham Crackers, Kellogg's Corn Flakes & American Health History / John Money*. Prometheus Books; 1985.

24 Banta, Jim E., Jerry W. Lee, Georgia Hodgkin, Zane Yi, Andrea Fanica, and Joan Sabate. 2018. "The Global Influence of the Seventh-Day Adventist Church on Diet." *Religions* 9, no. 9: 251.

25 Banta, Jim E., Jerry W. Lee, Georgia Hodgkin, Zane Yi, Andrea Fanica, and Joan Sabate. 2018. "The Global Influence of the Seventh-Day Adventist Church on Diet." *Religions* 9, no. 9: 251.

26 "Female Circumcision and Clitoridectomy in the United States: A History of a Medical Treatment." Journal of American History, Volume 102, Issue 2, September 2015, Pages 517–518.

27 https://australianfoodtimeline.com.au/muesli-invente/. Accessed December 19, 2023.

28 https://en.wikipedia.org/wiki/Lebensreform#:~:text=Representatives of the Lebensreform propagated,changes in the 19th century. Accessed December 19, 2023

29 Ibid.

30 Ibid.

31 James Gregory. *Of Victorians and Vegetarians: The Vegetarian Movement in Nineteenth-Century Britain*. London: Tauris Academic Studies, 2007

32 Weeks, J. (2017). *Sex, Politics and Society: The Regulation of Sexuality Since 1800* (4th ed.). Routledge.

33 https://www.rte.ie/history/post-famine/2020/0914/1165099-how-the-irish-famine-changed-new-york-city-forever/#:~:text=In the decade following the,of the city's total population. Accessed December 19, 2023.

34 https://www.loc.gov/classroom-materials/immigration/italian/the-great-arrival/. Accessed December 19, 2023.

35 Stone, Pamela, Shapiro Sanders Lise. *Bodies and Lives Victorian England: Science, Sexuality, and the Affliction of Being Female*. London: Routledge 2020.

36 Marland, H, *Health and Girlhood in Britain, 1874-1920*, London: Palgrave Macmillan, 2013.

37 Ibid.

38 James Gregory. *Of Victorians and Vegetarians: The Vegetarian Movement in Nineteenth-Century Britain*. London: Tauris Academic Studies, 2007.

39 Stone, Pamela, Shapiro Sanders Lise Bodies and Lives Victorian England: Science, Sexuality, and the Affliction of Being Female. London: Routledge 2020.

40 https://christiestratos.com/why-did-victorians-think-dangerous-women-read-novels-newspapers/. Accessed December 20, 2023.

41 https://christiestratos.com/why-did-victorians-think-dangerous-women-read-novels-newspapers/

42 Marland, H, *Health and Girlhood in Britain, 1874-1920*. London: Palgrave Macmillan, 2013.

43 Tasca C, Rapetti M, Carta MG, Fadda B. "Women and Hysteria in the History of Mental Health." *Clin Pract Epidemiol Ment Health*. 2012;8:110-9.

44 Weeks, J. (2017). *Sex, Politics and Society: The Regulation of Sexuality Since 1800* (4th ed.). Routledge.

45 Nathanson, C. *Dangerous Passage: The Social Control of Sexuality in Women's Adolescence*. Philadelphia: Temple University Press, 1991, 286.

46 Ibid.

47 https://www.irishtimes.com/news/social-affairs/mother-and-baby-homes-report-9-000-children-died-amid-high-infant-mortality-rate-1.4456382. Accessed December 19, 2023.

48 Rodriguez, Sarah B. *Female Circumcision and Clitoridectomy in the United States: A History of a Medical Treatment*. Boydell & Brewer, 2014.

49 Dwyer, E. *A Historical Perspective Sex Roles and Psychopathology*. pp. 19-38

50 Ibid.

51 Ibid.

52 Ibid.

53 T. Schlich. *Controlled Intervention: The History of Modern Surgery, 1800-1914*.

54 https://books.openedition.org/psorbonne/51471?lang=en. Accessed December 20, 2023.

55 Weeks, J. (2017). *Sex, Politics and Society: The Regulation of Sexuality Since 1800* (4th ed.). Routledge.

56 Ibid.

57 Marland, H. (2013). "Unstable Adolescence: Medicine and the 'Perils of Puberty' in Late Victorian and Edwardian Britain." In: *Health and Girlhood in Britain, 1874–1920. Palgrave Studies in the History of Childhood.* Palgrave Macmillan, London.

58 Bright, E. *Good Fat is Good for Women: Menopause*

59 Ibid.

60 J. B. Fleming. "Clitoridectomy -- The Disastrous Downfall of Isaac Baker Brown." *The Journal of Obstetrics and Gynaecology of the British Empire.* vol. 67, n. 6, 1960, p. 1018.

61 61. Rodriguez, Sarah B. *Female Circumcision and Clitoridectomy in the United States: A History of a Medical Treatment.* Boydell & Brewer, 2014.

62 Weeks, J. (2017). *Sex, Politics and Society: The Regulation of Sexuality Since 1800* (4th ed.). Routledge.

63 Hall, G. S., *Youth, Its Regimen and Hygiene.* New York: Appleton 1907.

64 Marland, H. *Health and Girlhood in Britain, 1874-1920.* London: Palgrave Macmillan, 2013.

65 Foucault, Michel, 1926-1984 author. *The History of Sexuality.* New York: Pantheon Books, 19782021.

66 Marland, H. *Health and Girlhood in Britain, 1874-1920.* London: Palgrave Macmillan, 2013.

67 Stone, Pamela, Shapiro Sanders Lise. *Bodies and Lives Victorian England: Science, Sexuality, and the Affliction of Being Female.* London: Routledge 2020.

68 Rayner JA, Pyett P, Astbury J. "The Medicalization of 'Tall' Girls: A Discourse Analysis of Medical Literature on the Use of Synthetic Oestrogen to Reduce Female Height." *Soc Sci Med.* 2010 Sep;71(6):1076-83.

69 Jumana, Rumaisa Nasim, "Mental Illness and Psychiatry in the Victorian Era: An Analysis of the Prevailing Power Dynamics Between Women and Male Authority Figures Through Gilman and Freud." (2019). *CUNY Academic Works.*

70 Donkin, Horatio Bryan. *Hysteria: A Dictionary of Psychological Medicine with the Symptoms, Treatment and Pathology of Insanity and the Law of Lunacy in Great Britain and Ireland.* Ed. Daniel Hack Tuke. London: Churchill, 1892. 618–27.

71 Marland, H. (2013). "Unstable Adolescence: Medicine and the 'Perils of Puberty' in Late Victorian and Edwardian Britain." In: *Health and Girlhood in Britain, 1874–1920. Palgrave Studies in the History of Childhood.* Palgrave Macmillan, London.

72 Biller J G. "Treatment of Neurasthenia." *JAMA.* 1902;XXXVIII(1):4–6.

73 Lasègue, Ernest-Charles. "De l'anorexie hystérique." *Journal Français de Psychiatrie*, vol. 32, no. 1, 2009, pp. 3-8.

74 Brumberg, Joan Jacobs. *The Fasting Girls.* New York, NY: Plume, 1989

75 Bruch H. *The Golden Cage.* Harvard University Press 1978

76 Brumberg, Joan Jacobs. *The Fasting Girls.* New York, NY: Plume, 1989

77 Ibid.

78 Brumberg JJ. "Chlorotic Girls, 1870-1920: A Historical Perspective on Female Adolescence." *Child Dev.* 1982 Dec;53(6):1468-77

79 https://www.researchgate.net/publication 265264616_Feminist_Food_Studies_A_Brief_History

80 https://en.wikipedia.org/wiki/Warnaco_Group. Accessed December 16, 2023

81 Dwyer, E. (1984). "A Historical Perspective." In: Widom, C.S. (eds) *Sex Roles and Psychopathology.* Springer, Boston, MA.

82 Brumberg, Joan Jacobs. *The Fasting Girls.* New York, NY: Plume, 1989

83 Ibid

84 J. B. Fleming. "Clitoridectomy -- The Disastrous Downfall of Isaac Baker Brown." *The Journal of Obstetrics and Gynaecology of the British Empire.* vol. 67, n. 6, 1960, p. 1018.

85 Rodriguez, Sarah B. *Female Circumcision and Clitoridectomy in the United States: A History of a Medical Treatment.* Boydell & Brewer, 2014.

THREE
WHAT IS PUBERTY?

1 Muuss R E. *Theories of Adolescence.* New York: McGraw Hill, 1996.

2 Angold, A., Costello, E., and Worthman, C. (1998). "Puberty and Depression: The Roles of Age, Pubertal Status and Pubertal Timing." *Psychological Medicine*, 28(1), 51-61.

3 Torabinejad S, Miro C, Barone B, Imbimbo C, Crocetto F, Dentice M. "The Androgen-Thyroid Hormone Crosstalk in Prostate Cancer and the Clinical Implications." *Eur Thyroid J.* 2023 Apr 26;12(3):e220228

4 Gregorasczuk EL, Kolodziejczyk J, Rzysa J. "Triiodothyronine Stimulates 3Beta-Hydroxysteroid Dehydrogenase Activity in the Porcine Corpus Luteum." *Endocr Regul.* 1999 Dec;33(4):155.

5 Weber G, Vigone MC, Stroppa L, Chiumello G. "Thyroid Function and Puberty." *J Pediatr Endocrinol Metab.* 2003 Mar;16 Suppl 2:253-7.

6 Wang Y, He D, Fu C, Dong X, Jiang F, Su M, Xu Q, Huang P, Wang N, Chen Y, Jiang Q. "Thyroid Function Changes and Pubertal Progress in Females: A Longitudinal Study in Iodine-Sufficient Areas of East China." *Front Endocrinol* (Lausanne). 2021 May 11;12:653680

7 Emmanuel M, Bokor BR. *Tanner Stages.* [Updated 2022 Dec 11]. In: StatPearls [Internet]. Treasure Island (FL): StatPearls Publishing; 2023 Jan-

8 Biro FM, Huang B, Daniels SR, Lucky AW. "Pubarche as well as Thelarche may be a Marker for the Onset of Puberty." *J Pediatr Adolesc Gynecol.* 2008 Dec;21(6):323-8.

9 Emmanuel M, Bokor BR. *Tanner Stages.* [Updated 2022 Dec 11]. In: StatPearls [Internet]. Treasure Island (FL): StatPearls Publishing; 2023 Jan-

10 Langston, Nancy. *Toxic Bodies: Hormone Disruptors and the Legacy of DES.* Yale University Press, 2010. ec. 2023.

11 Michaud P, Foradori A, Rodríguez-Portales JA, Arteaga E, López JM, Téllez R. "A Prepubertal Surge of Thyrotropin Precedes an Increase in Thyroxine and 3,5,3'-Triiodothyronine in Normal Children." *J Clin Endocrinol Metab.* 1991 May;72(5):976-81.

12 Emmanuel M, Bokor BR. *Tanner Stages.* 2022 Dec 11. In: StatPearls [Internet]. Treasure Island (FL): StatPearls Publishing; 2023 Jan–

13 Biro FM, Huang B, Daniels SR, Lucky AW. "Pubarche as well as Thelarche may be a Marker for the Onset of Puberty." *J Pediatr Adolesc Gynecol.* 2008 Dec;21(6):323-8.

14 https://www.smh.com.au/lifestyle/health-and-wellness/get-cliterate-how-a-melbourne-doctor-is-redefining-female-sexuality-20181203-p50jvv.html. Accessed December 15, 2023.

15 https://www.nytimes.com/2022/10/17/health/clitoris-sex-doctors-surgery.html. Accessed December 2, 2023.

16 Langston, Nancy. *Toxic Bodies: Hormone Disruptors and the Legacy of DES.* Yale University Press, 2010. ec. 2023.

17 Shankar Kikkeri N, Nagalli S. *Turner Syndrome.* [Updated 2023 Aug 8]. In: StatPearls [Internet]. Treasure Island (FL): StatPearls Publishing; 2023 Jan-.

18 https://medium.com/canzoni-in-una-stanza/not-a-love-song-women-who-dont-sing-about-love-27ffbe19f2d2. Accessed December 18.

19 https://www.nytimes.com/interactive/2023/08/09/magazine/female-rappers.html. Accessed December 18.

20 https://www.nytimes.com/interactive/2023/08/09/magazine/female-rappers.html. Accessed December 18.

FOUR
THE CAUSES OF HEALTH ISSUES DURING PUBERTY

1 Michaud P, Foradori A, Rodríguez-Portales JA, Arteaga E, López JM, Téllez R. "A Prepubertal Surge of Thyrotropin Precedes an Increase in Thyroxine and 3,5,3'-Triiodothyronine in Normal Children. *J Clin Endocrinol Metab*. 1991 May;72(5):976-81.

2 Zhou Q, Xue S, Zhang L, Chen G. "Trace Elements and the Thyroid." *Front Endocrinol* (Lausanne). 2022 Oct 24;13:904889. doi: 10.3389/fendo.2022.904889.

3 Krishnamurthy HK, Reddy S, Jayaraman V, Krishna K, Song Q, Rajasekaran KE, Wang T, Bei K, Rajasekaran JJ. "Effect of Micronutrients on Thyroid Parameters." *J Thyroid Res*. 2021 Sep 28;2021:1865483.

4 Ibid.

5 Ibid.

6 Ibid.

7 Triggiani V, Tafaro E, Giagulli VA, Sabbà C, Resta F, Licchelli B, Guastamacchia E. "Role of Iodine, Selenium and Other Micronutrients in Thyroid Function and Disorders." *Endocr Metab Immune Disord Drug Targets*. 2009 Sep;9(3):277-94.

8 Marine D, Baumann EJ, Cipra A. "Studies on Simple Goiter Produced by Cabbage and Other Vegetables." *Proceedings of the Society for Experimental Biology and Medicine*. 1929;26(9):822-824

9 Marine D. "Prevention and Treatment of Simple Goiter." *Atl. Med. J.*, 26:437-442, 1923.

10 Diosady LL, Alberti JO, Ramcharan K, Mannar MG. "Iodine Stability in Salt Double-Fortified with Iron and Iodine." *Food Nutr Bull*. 2002 Jun;23(2):196-207.

11 Salter, W.T. *The Endocrine Function of Iodine*. Harvard University Press, 1940, Cambridge, Mass., pg 254-255, 261, 268-269.

12 Abraham, G.E., Flechas, J.D., Hakala, J.C. "Optimum Levels of Iodine for Greatest Mental and Physical Health." *The Original Internist* 9:5-20, 2002

13 Parry CH. *Collections from the Unpublished Medical Writings of* C. H. *Parry*. London, Underwoods 1825; 2: 11-128.

14 Huang HB, Cheng PK, Siao CY, Lo YC, Chou WC, Huang PC. "Mediation Effects of Thyroid Function in the Associations between Phthalate Exposure and Lipid Metabolism in Adults." *Environ Health.* 2022 Jul 1;21(1):61.

15 Vitti, Paolo; Hegedüs, Laszlo (2018). [Endocrinology] *Thyroid Diseases: Drugs and Other Substances Interfering with Thyroid Function.*

16 Giuliani C, Bucci I, Di Santo S, Rossi C, Grassadonia A, Piantelli M, Monaco F, Napolitano G. "The Flavonoid Quercetin Inhibits Thyroid-Restricted Genes Expression and Thyroid Function." *Food Chem Toxicol.* 2014 Apr;66:23-9.

17 Dong BJ. "How Medications Affect Thyroid Function." West J Med. 2000 Feb;172(2):102-6.

18 Yıldırım N, Doğan S, Atakan N. "Evaluation of Thyroid Function Tests of Acne Vulgaris Patients Treated with Systemic Isotretinoin." *J Dermatolog Treat.* 2017 Mar;28(2):141-144

19 Caye, Arthur; Pilz, Luisa K.; Maia, Ana L.; Hidalgo, Maria Paz; Furukawa, Toshi A.; Kieling, Christian (2020). "The Impact of Selective Serotonin Reuptake Inhibitors on the Thyroid Function among Patients with Major Depressive Disorder: A Systematic Review and Meta-Analysis." *European Neuropsychopharmacology* (), S0924977X20300341–.

20 Pisano S, Pozzi M, Catone G, Scrinzi G, Clementi E, Coppola G, Milone A, Bravaccio C, Santosh P, Masi G. "Putative Mechanisms of Action and Clinical Use of Lithium in Children and Adolescents: A Critical Review." *Curr Neuropharmacol.* 2019;17(4):318-341.

21 Vitti, Paolo; Hegedüs, Laszlo (2018). [Endocrinology] "Thyroid Diseases: Drugs and Other Substances Interfering with Thyroid Function."

22 Jerome M. Hershman. "The Role of Human Chorionic Gonadotropin as a Thyroid Stimulator in Normal Pregnancy." The Journal of Clinical Endocrinology & Metabolism, Volume 93, Issue 9, 1 September 2008, Pages 3305–3306

23 https://www.bestbuyhcg.com/modified-800-calorie-hcg-like-diet-older-teens/. Accessed December 18 2023.

24 Man EB, Shaver BA, Cooke RE: "Studies of Children Born to Women with Thyroid Disease." *Am J Obstet Gynecol* 1958; 75: 728.

25 Abraham, G.E. "The Wolff-Chaikoff Effect: Crying Wolf?" *The Original Internist*, 12(3):112-118, 2005.

26 Delange F. "Iodine Deficiency in Europe and its Consequences: An Update." *Eur J Nucl Med Mol Imaging*. 2002 Aug;29 Suppl 2:S404-16.

27 Wang Y, He D, Fu C, Dong X, Jiang F, Su M, Xu Q, Huang P, Wang N, Chen Y, Jiang Q. "Thyroid Function Changes and Pubertal Progress in Females: A Longitudinal Study in Iodine-Sufficient Areas of East China." *Front Endocrinol* (Lausanne). 2021 May 11;12:653680.

28 Velasco I, Rueda-Etxebarria M, Trak-Fellermeier MA, Taylor P, Rabassa Bonet M, Rueda JR, Chi Y, Janka H. "Iodine Supplementation for Preventing Iodine Deficiency Disorders in Children and Adolescents." *Cochrane Database Syst Rev*. 2023 Apr 28;2023(4):CD014475

29 Salter, W.T. *The Endocrine Function of Iodine*. Harvard University Press, 1940, Cambridge, Mass., pg 254-255, 261, 268-269.

30 Ghent WR, Eskin BA, Low DA, Hill LP. "Iodine Replacement in Fibrocystic Disease of the Breast." *Can J Surg*. 1993 Oct;36(5):453-60.

31 Ramsden CE, Zamora D, Majchrzak-Hong S, Faurot KR, Broste SK, Frantz RP, Davis JM, Ringel A, Suchindran CM, Hibbeln JR. "Re-Evaluation of the Traditional Diet-Heart Hypothesis: Analysis of Recovered Data from Minnesota Coronary Experiment (1968-73)." *BMJ*. 2016 Apr 12;353:i1246.

32 Joffe, Russell T., 1954- and Levitt, Anthony J., 1959-. *The Thyroid Axis and Psychiatric Illness*. edited by Russell T. Joffe, Anthony J. Levitt American Psychiatric Press Washington, DC 1993.

33 Miller WL, Bose HS. "Early Steps in Steroidogenesis: Intracellular Cholesterol Trafficking." *J Lipid Res*. 2011 Dec;52(12):2111-2135.

34 Kota AS, Ejaz S. *Precocious Puberty*. [Updated 2023 Jul 4]. In: StatPearls [Internet]. Treasure Island (FL): StatPearls Publishing; 2023 Jan-.

35 Holst JP, Soldin OP, Guo T, Soldin SJ. "Steroid Hormones: Relevance and Measurement in the Clinical Laboratory." *Clin Lab Med*. 2004 Mar;24(1):105-18.

36 Gibb FW, Homer NZ, Faqehi AM, Upreti R, Livingstone DE, McInnes KJ, Andrew R, Walker BR. "Aromatase Inhibition Reduces Insulin Sensitivity in Healthy Men." *J Clin Endocrinol Metab*. 2016 May;101(5):2040-6.

37 McTernan, Philip G.; Anderson, Leah A.; Anwar, Aresh J.; Eggo, Margaret C.; Crocker, John; Barnett, Anthony H.; Stewart, Paul M.; Kumar, Sudhesh (2002). "Glucocorticoid Regulation of P450 Aromatase Activity in Human Adipose Tissue: Gender and Site Differences." *The Journal of Clinical Endocrinology & Metabolism*, 87(3), 1327–1336.

38 Morey JN, Boggero IA, Scott AB, Segerstrom SC. "Current Directions in Stress and Human Immune Function." *Curr Opin Psychol.* 2015 Oct 1;5:13-17.

39 Banta, Jim E., Jerry W. Lee, Georgia Hodgkin, Zane Yi, Andrea Fanica, and Joan Sabate. 2018. "The Global Influence of the Seventh-Day Adventist Church on Diet." *Religions* 9, no. 9: 251.

40 Ibid.

41 Banta, Jim E., Jerry W. Lee, Georgia Hodgkin, Zane Yi, Andrea Fanica, and Joan Sabate. 2018. "The Global Influence of the Seventh-Day Adventist Church on Diet." *Religions* 9, no. 9: 251.

42 https://www.vndpg.org/about/academy-co-founder-lenna-frances-cooper-a-pioneer-in-vegetarian-nutrition-and-dietetics.

43 Yudkin, John, 1910-1995. *Pure, White and Deadly: the Problem of Sugar.* London :Davis-Poynter Ltd, 1972.

44 https://www.scientificamerican.com/article/records-found-in-dusty-basement-undermine-decades-of-dietary-advice/.

45 Meach R. From John Yudkin to Jamie Oliver: *A Short but Sweet History on the War against Sugar.* In: Gentilcore D, Smith M, editors. Proteins, Pathologies and Politics: Dietary Innovation and Disease from the Nineteenth Century. London (UK); New York (NY): Bloomsbury Academic; 2018. Chapter 7.

46 https://www.latimes.com/archives/la-xpm-1985-03-01-mn-23924-story.html. Accessed December 23, 2023.

47 https://www.ministrymagazine.org/archive/1978/04/nutrition-and-health. Accessed December 23, 2023.

48 https://isupportgary.com/uploads/articles/McGovern-Report-Pritikin-Adventist-www.isupportgary.com.pdf. Accessed December 23, 2023.

49 Morton, D.; Rankin, P.; Kent, L.; Dysinger, W. (2016). "The Complete Health Improvement Program (CHIP): History, Evaluation, and Outcomes." *American Journal of Lifestyle Medicine*, 10(1), 64–73.

50 Gregg, E. W.; Cadwell, B. L.; Cheng, Y. J.; Cowie, C. C.; Williams, D. E.; Geiss, L.; Engelgau, M. M.; Vinicor, F. (2004). "Trends in the Prevalence and Ratio of Diagnosed to Undiagnosed Diabetes According to Obesity Levels in the U.S." *Diabetes Care*, 27(12), 2806–2812.

51 GBD 2021 Diabetes Collaborators. "Global, Regional, and National Burden of Diabetes from 1990 to 2021, with Projections of Prevalence to 2050: A Systematic Analysis for the Global Burden of Disease Study 2021." *Lancet.* 2023 Jul 15;402(10397):203-234.

52 Steele, S., Ruskin, G., Sarcevic, L. *et al.* "Are Industry-Funded Charities Promoting ‹Advocacy-led Studies' or ‹Evidence-Based Science?: A Case Study of the International Life Sciences Institute." *Global Health* **15**, 36 (2019). https://doi.org/10.1186/s12992-019-0478-6

53 Banta, Jim E., Jerry W. Lee, Georgia Hodgkin, Zane Yi, Andrea Fanica, and Joan Sabate. 2018. "The Global Influence of the Seventh-Day Adventist Church on Diet." *Religions* 9, no. 9: 251.

54 Swim, Janet K., Theresa K. Vescio, Julia L. Dahl, and Stephanie J. Zawadzki. 2018. "Gendered Discourse About Climate Change Policies." *Global Environmental Change* 48: 216–25.

55 https://en.wikipedia.org/wiki/Hypatia#:~:text=Hypatia (born c. 350– ,she taught philosophy and astronomy. Accessed December 23, 2023.

56 Langston, Nancy. *Toxic Bodies: Hormone Disruptors and the Legacy of DES.* Yale University Press, 2010. ec. 2023.

57 Bright, E. *Good Fat is Good for Women: Menopause.*

FIVE
MEDICINES FOR PUBERTY

1 Bright E, *Good Fat Is Good For Women: Menopause*

2 Vertinsky P. "Exercise, Physical Capability, and the Eternally Wounded Woman in Late Nineteenth Century North America." *J Sport Hist.* 1987;14(1):7-2.

3 Clarke, Edward H. *Sex In Education or A Fair Chance For The Girls.* Houghton, Mifflin, and Co., 1873.

4 Maudsley, Henry. "Sex In Mind And in Education." *Popular Science Monthly* volume 5, June 1874 https://en.wikisource.org/wiki/Popular_Science_Monthly/Volume_5/June_1874/Sex_in_Mind_and_Education. Accessed December 22, 2023.

5 Yazici E, Bursalioglu FS, Aydin N, Yazici AB. "Menarche, Puberty and Psychiatric Disorders." *Gynecol Endocrinol.* 2013 Dec;29(12):1055-8. doi: 10.3109/09513590.2013.829447. Epub 2013 Aug 23.

6 Dwyer. *A Historical Perspective.* Springer US, 1984.

7 https://www.independent.co.uk/news/health/labiaplasty-vagina-surgery-cosmetic-procedure-plastic-study-international-society-aesthetic-plastic-surgeons-usa-a7837181.html. Accessed December 20, 2023.

8 Ginger VA, Cold CJ, Yang CC. "Surgical Anatomy of the Dorsal Nerve of the Clitoris." *Neurourol Urodyn.* 2011 Mar;30(3):412-6

9 Rodriguez, Sarah B. *Female Circumcision and Clitoridectomy in the United States: A History of a Medical Treatment.*

10 https://www.stephenmchen.com/post/why-is-labiaplasty-on-the-rise. Accessed December 20, 2023

11 Clerico, C.; Lari, A.; Mojallal, A.; Boucher, F. (2017). "Anatomy and Aesthetics of the Labia Minora: The Ideal Vulva?" *Aesthetic Plastic Surgery*, 41(3), 714–719.

12 Belloli G, Campobasso P, Musi L. "Labial Skin-Flap Vaginoplasty Using Tissue Expanders." *Pediatr Surg Int.* 1997 Feb;12(2-3):168-71.

13 Ndoye, M., Gueye, S., Niang, L., Cassim, F., Adlam, J. (2023). "Female Genital Mutilation/Cutting." In: Martins, F.E., Holm, H.V., Sandhu, J.S., McCammon, K.A. (eds) *Female Genitourinary and Pelvic Floor Reconstruction.* Springer, Cham.

14 https://www.nytimes.com/2022/10/17/health/clitoris-sex-doctors-surgery.html. Accessed December 20, 2023.

15 Rodriguez, Sarah B. *Female Circumcision and Clitoridectomy in the United States: A History of a Medical Treatment.*

16 Ibid.

17 Ibid.

18 Ibid.

19 Ibid.

20 H. M. Behre [et al.]. "Efficency and Safety of an Injectable Combination Hormonal Contraceptive for Men." *Journal of Clinical Endocrinology & Metabolism.* vol. 101, n. 12, 2016, p. 4779-4788.

21 B. Squires. "The Racist and Sexist History of Keeping Birth Control Side Effects Secret." *Vice* October 17, 2016, https://broadly.vice.com/en_us/article/kzeazz/the-racist-and-sexist-history-of-keeping-birth-control-side-effects-secret, accessed 23 December 2018.

22 Shostak, Marjorie. *Nisa: The Life and Words of a !Kung Woman.* Harvard University Press, 1981.

23 Kilberg MJ, Vogiatzi MG. "Approach to the Patient: Central Precocious Puberty." *J Clin Endocrinol Metab.* 2023 Jul 14;108(8):2115-2123.

24 Martinez GM. "Trends and Patterns in Menarche in the United States: 1995 through 2013-2017." *Natl Health Stat Report.* 2020 Sep;(146):1-12

25 Lee JE, Jung HW, Lee YJ, Lee YA. "Early-Life Exposure to Endocrine-Disrupting Chemicals and Pubertal Development in Girls." *Ann Pediatr Endocrinol Metab.* 2019 Jun;24(2):78-91.

26 Euling SY, Selevan SG, Pescovitz OH, Skakkebaek NE. "Role of Environmental Factors in the Timing of Puberty." *Pediatrics*. 2008 Feb;121 Suppl 3:S167-71.

27 Herman-Giddens ME, Slora EJ, Wasserman RC, Bourdony CJ, Bhapkar MV, Koch GG, Hasemeier CM. "Secondary Sexual Characteristics and Menses in Young Girls seen in Office Practice: A Study from the Pediatric Research in Office Settings Network." *Pediatrics*. 1997 Apr;99(4):505-12.

28 Yaşa C, Güngör Uğurlucan F. "Approach to Abnormal Uterine Bleeding in Adolescents." *J Clin Res Pediatr Endocrinol*. 2020 Feb 6;12(Suppl 1):1-6.

29 Herman-Giddens ME, Slora EJ, Wasserman RC, Bourdony CJ, Bhapkar MV, Koch GG, Hasemeier CM. "Secondary Sexual Characteristics and Menses in Young Girls seen in Office Practice: A Study from the Pediatric Research in Office Settings Network." *Pediatrics*. 1997 Apr;99(4):505-12.

30 Park SE, Ahn JY, Kim EY. "The Assessment of Brain Volume Differences in Idiopathic Central Precocious Puberty Girls; Comparison of Age-Matched Girls and Normal Puberty Girls." *Children* (Basel). 2021 Sep 11;8(9):797.

31 Mendle J, Moore SR, Briley DA, Harden KP. "Puberty, Socioeconomic Status, and Depression in Girls: Evidence for Gene × Environment Interactions." *Clin Psychol Sci*. 2016 Jan 1;4(1):3-16.

32 Bräuner EV, Busch AS, Eckert-Lind C, Koch T, Hickey M, Juul A. "Trends in the Incidence of Central Precocious Puberty and Normal Variant Puberty Among Children in Denmark, 1998 to 2017." *JAMA Netw Open*. 2020 Oct 1;3(10):e2015665.

33 McGuire TC, McCormick KC, Koch MK, Mendle J. "Pubertal Maturation and Trajectories of Depression During Early Adolescence." *Front Psychol*. 2019 Jun 12;10:1362.

34 https://www.nytimes.com/2022/01/20/well/sustainable-period-products.html. Accessed December 23. 2023.

35 https://www.popsci.com/story/health/pfas-period-underwear-toxic-chemicals/. Accessed December 23, 2023.

36 https://www.ehn.org/pfas-tampons-2658510849.html. Accessed December 23, 2023.

37 Graber, Julia. (2013). "Pubertal Timing and the Development of Psychopathology in Adolescence and Beyond." *Hormones and Behavior*. 64. 262-9. 10.1016/j.yhbeh.2013.04.003.

38 https://www.apa.org/monitor/2016/03/puberty. Accessed December 23, 2023.

39 Ibid.

40 Ibid.

41 Ornella Moscucci. *The Science of Woman: Gynaecology and Gender in England, 1800-1929.* Cambridge University Press, 1990.

42 Wheeler, M.D., Styne, D.M. "Drug Treatment in Precocious Puberty." *Drugs* 41, 717–728 (1991).

43 De Sanctis V, Soliman AT, Di Maio S, Soliman N, Elsedfy H. "Long-Term Effects and Significant Adverse Drug Reactions (ADRs) Associated with the Use of Gonadotropin-Releasing Hormone Analogs (GnRHa) for Central Precocious Puberty: A Brief Review of Literature." *Acta Biomed.* 2019 Sep 6;90(3):345-359.

44 Saggese G, Bertelloni S, Baroncelli GI, Battini R, Franchi G. "Reduction of Bone Density: An Effect of Gonadotropin Releasing Hormone Analogue Treatment in Central Precocious Puberty." *Eur J Pediatr.* 1993 Sep;152(9):717-20.

45 Klein KO, Barnes KM, Jones JV, Feuillan PP, Cutler GB Jr. "Increased Final Height in Precocious Puberty after Long-Term Treatment with LHRH Agonists: The National Institutes of Health Experience." *J Clin Endocrinol Metab.* 2001 Oct;86(10):4711-6.

46 McCartney CR, Campbell RE, Marshall JC, Moenter SM. "The Role of Gonadotropin-Releasing Hormone Neurons in Polycystic Ovary Syndrome." *J Neuroendocrinol.* 2022; 34:e13093

47 De Sanctis V, Soliman AT, Di Maio S, Soliman N, Elsedfy H. "Long-Term Effects and Significant Adverse Drug Reactions (ADRs) Associated with the Use of Gonadotropin-Releasing Hormone Analogs (GnRHa) for Central Precocious Puberty: A Brief Review of Literature." *Acta Biomed.* 2019 Sep 6;90(3):345-359.

48 Ibid.

49 Ibid.

50 Klein KO, Barnes KM, Jones JV, Feuillan PP, Cutler GB Jr. "Increased Final Height in Precocious Puberty after Long-Term Treatment with LHRH Agonists: The National Institutes of Health Experience." *J Clin Endocrinol Metab.* 2001 Oct;86(10):4711-6

51 Franzini IA, Yamamoto FM, Bolfi F, Antonini SR, Nunes-Nogueira VS. "GnRH Analog is Ineffective in Increasing Adult Height in Girls with Puberty Onset after 7 Years of Age: A Systematic Review and Meta-Analysis." *Eur J Endocrinol.* 2018 Dec 1;179(6):381-390.

52 Hoberman, J. (2005). *Testosterone Dreams: Rejuvenation, Aphrodisia, Doping*. Berkeley: University of California Press.

53 Rasmussen, N. "Of ` Small Men', Big Science and Bigger Business: The Second World War and Biomedical Research in the United States." *Minerva* 40, 115–146 (2002).

54 George MM, Eugster EA, Chernausek SD. *Pituitary Gigantism*. [Updated 2022 Jun 22]. In: Feingold KR, Anawalt B, Blackman MR, et al., editors. Endotext [Internet]. South Dartmouth (MA): MDText.com, Inc.; 2000-.

55 Rayner JA, Pyett P, Astbury J. "The Medicalization of 'Tall' Girls: A Discourse Analysis of Medical Literature on the Use of Synthetic Oestrogen to Reduce Female Height." *Soc Sci Med*. 2010 Sep;71(6):1076-8.

56 Ibid.

57 Ibid.

58 58. https://www.rxlist.com/how_do_gonadotropin_releasing_hormone_antagonists/drug-class.htm. Accessed December 23, 2023.

59 Yoon JY, Cheon CK. "Evaluation and Management of Amenorrhea Related to Congenital Sex Hormonal Disorders." *Ann Pediatr Endocrinol Metab*. 2019 Sep;24(3):149-157.

60 https://www.rxlist.com/clomid-drug.htm. Accessed December 23, 2023.

61 Yu O, Christ JP, Schulze-Rath R, Covey J, Kelley A, Grafton J, Cronkite D, Holden E, Hilpert J, Sacher F, Micks E, Reed SD. "Incidence, Prevalence, and Trends in Polycystic Ovary Syndrome Diagnosis: A United States Population-Based Study from 2006 to 2019." *Am J Obstet Gynecol*. 2023 Jul;229(1):39.e1-39.e12.

62 Zhao, H., Zhang, J., Cheng, X. et al. "Insulin Resistance in Polycystic Ovary Syndrome across Various Tissues: An Updated Review of Pathogenesis, Evaluation, and Treatment." *J Ovarian Res* 16, 9 (2023).

63 Wright PJ, Corbett CL, Pinto BM, Dawson RM, Wirth MD. "The Impact of Exercise Perceptions and Depressive Symptoms on Polycystic Ovary Syndrome–Specific Health-Related Quality of Life." *Women's Health*. 2021;17.

64 Buggs C, Rosenfield RL. "Polycystic Ovary Syndrome in Adolescence." *Endocrinol Metab Clin North Am*. 2005 Sep;34(3):677-705, x.

65 https://www.mayoclinic.org/drugs-supplements/metformin-oral-route/side-effects/drg-20067074. Accessed December 23, 2023.

66 https://www.mayoclinic.org/drugs-supplements/pioglitazone-oral-route/side-effects/

drg-20065503?p=1#:~:text=Descriptions,your body use insulin better. Accessed December 23, 2023.

67 Pai SA, Kshirsagar NA. "Pioglitazone Utilization, Efficacy & Safety in Indian Type 2 Diabetic Patients: A Systematic Review & Comparison with European Medicines Agency Assessment Report." *Indian J Med Res.* 2016 Nov;144(5):672-681.

68 https://www.mayoclinic.org/drugs-supplements/rosiglitazone-oral-route/side-effects/drg-20066965?p=1. Accessed December 23, 2023.

69 https://dfda.goa.gov.in/media-1/158-ban-on-manufacture-for-sale-and-distribution-of-rosiglitazone-and-their-formulations-for-human-use#:~:text=Government of India in excercise,immediate effect in the country.

70 https://www.mayoclinic.org/drugs-supplements/liraglutide-subcutaneous-route/side-effects/drg-20073828?p=1#:~:text=Check with your doctor right, and requires immediate medical attention. Accessed December 23, 2023.

71 https://www.mayoclinic.org/drugs-supplements/exenatide-subcutaneous-route/side-effects/drg-20068401.

72 https://www.mayoclinic.org/drugs-supplements/semaglutide-subcutaneous-route/side-effects/drg-20406730?p=1. Accessed December 23, 2023.

73 https://www.mayoclinic.org/drugs-supplements/sitagliptin-oral-route/side-effects/drg-20069730?p=1. Accessed December 23, 2023.

74 https://www.mayoclinic.org/drugs-supplements/dapagliflozin-oral-route/side-effects/drg-20095101. Accessed December 23, 2023.

75 https://www.mayoclinic.org/drugs-supplements/empagliflozin-oral-route/side-effects/drg-20113010?p=1. Accessed December 23, 2023.

76 https://www.mayoclinic.org/drugs-supplements/linagliptin-oral-route/side-effects/drg-20074875?p=1#:~:text=Check with your doctor right, taken together with certain medicines. Accessed December 23, 2023.

77 https://www.mayoclinic.org/drugs-supplements/canagliflozin-oral-route/side-effects/drg-20060957. Accessed December 23, 2023.

78 https://www.mayoclinic.org/drugs-supplements/prednisone-oral-route/side-effects/drg-20075269. Accessed December 23, 2023.

79 https://www.mayoclinic.org/drugs-supplements/dexamethasone-oral-route/side-effects/drg-20075207?p=1 Accessed December 23, 2023.

80 Bright E. *Good Fat Is Good For Women: Menopause*

81 Ibid.

82 Regidor P-A, Mueller A, Mayr M. "Pharmacological and Metabolic Effects of Drospirenone as a Progestin-Only Pill Compared to Combined Formulations with Estrogen." *Women's Health.* 2023;19.

83 Leroy C Folmar; Michael J Hemmer; Nancy D Denslow; Kevin Kroll; Jian Chen; Ann Cheek; Harold Richman; Hillary Meredith; E.Gordon Grau (2002). "A Comparison of the Estrogenic Potencies of Estradiol, Ethynylestradiol, Diethylstilbestrol, Nonylphenol and Methoxychlor in Vivo and in Vitro. , 60(1-2), 0–110.

84 Bright E. *Good Fat Is Good For Women: Menopause.*

85 Ibid.

86 Ibid

87 Seaman B. The Greatest Experiment Ever Performed on Women. New York: Seven Stories Press, 2011.

88 Christopher Tietze (1979). "The Pill and Mortality from Cardiovascular Disease: Another Look." *Family Planning Perspectives,* 11(2), 80–84.

89 Gillum LA, Mamidipudi SK, Johnston SC. "Ischemic Stroke Risk with Oral Contraceptives: A Meta-Analysis." *JAMA.* 2000 Jul 5;284(1):72-8.

90 Asthana S, Busa V, Labani S. "Oral Contraceptives Use and Risk of Cervical Cancer-A Systematic Review & Meta-Analysis." *Eur J Obstet Gynecol Reprod Biol.* 2020 Apr;247:163-175.

91 Godsland IF, Walton C, Felton C, Proudler A, Patel A, Wynn V. "Insulin Resistance, Secretion, and Metabolism in Users of Oral Contraceptives." *J Clin Endocrinol Metab.* 1992 Jan;74(1):64-70

92 Seaman B. The Greatest Experiment Ever Performed on Women. New York: Seven Stories Press, 2011.

93 Ibid.

94 Hughes LD, Majekodunmi O. "Hormonal Contraception and Suicide: A New Dimension of Risk." *Br J Gen Pract.* 2018 Nov;68(676):512-513.

95 Skovlund CW, Mørch LS, Kessing LV, Lidegaard Ø. "Association of Hormonal Contraception With Depression." *JAMA Psychiatry.* 2016 Nov 1;73(11):1154-1162.

96 Williams H. *Pregnant Or Dead: The Pill in New Perspective.* New Perspectives Publication, 1969.

97 Johansson T, Vinther Larsen S, Bui M, Ek WE, Karlsson T, Johansson Å. "Population-Based Cohort Study of Oral Contraceptive Use and Risk of Depression." *Epidemiol Psychiatr Sci.* 2023 Jun 12;32:e39.

98 Torre F, Calogero AE, Condorelli RA, Cannarella R, Aversa A, La Vignera S. "Effects of Oral Contraceptives on Thyroid Function and Vice Versa." *J Endocrinol Invest.* 2020 Sep;43(9):1181-1188.

99 Myasoedova E, Crowson CS, Kremers HM, Therneau TM, Gabriel SE. "Is the Incidence of Rheumatoid Arthritis Rising? Results from Olmsted County, Minnesota, 1955-2007." *Arthritis Rheum.* 2010 Jun;62(6):1576-82.

100 Shreenath AP, Kahloon A. Hepatic Adenoma. [Updated 2023 Jan 16]. In: StatPearls [Internet]. Treasure Island (FL): StatPearls Publishing; 2023 Jan-.

101 Thijs C, Knipschild P. "Oral Contraceptives and the Risk of Gallbladder Disease: A Meta-Analysis." *Am J Public Health.* 1993 Aug;83(8):1113-20.

102 https://www.health.harvard.edu/blog/astounding-increase-in-antidepressant-use-by-americans-201110203624. Accessed December 23, 2023.

103 Coupland C, Hill T, Morriss R, Arthur A, Moore M, Hippisley-Cox J. "Antidepressant Use and Risk of Suicide and Attempted Suicide or Self-Harm in People Aged 20 to 64: Cohort Study Using a Primary Care Database." *BMJ.* 2015 Feb 18;350:h517.

104 https://www.mayoclinic.org/diseases-conditions/depression/in-depth/ssris/art-20044825. Accessed December 23, 2023.

105 https://www.mayoclinic.org/drugs-supplements/gabapentin-oral-route/side-effects/drg-20064011?p=1. Accessed December 23, 2023.

106 https://www.mayoclinic.org/drugs-supplements/alprazolam-oral-route/side-effects/drg-20061040?p=1. Accessed December 23. 2023.

107 Persson, P., Qiu, X., & Rossin-Slater, M. (2021). "Family Spillover Effects of Marginal Diagnoses: The Case of ADHD."

108 Kok FM, Groen Y, Fuermaier ABM, Tucha O. "The Female Side of Pharmacotherapy for ADHD-A Systematic Literature Review." *PLoS One.* 2020 Sep 18;15(9):e0239257.

109 Haimov-Kochman R, Berger I. "Cognitive Functions of Regularly Cycling Women May Differ Throughout the Month, Depending on Sex Hormone Status; A Possible Explanation to Conflicting Results of Studies of ADHD in Females." *Front Hum Neurosci.* 2014 Apr 1;8:191.

110 Lasègue, Ernest-Charles. "De l'anorexie hystérique." *Journal Français de Psychiatrie*, vol. 32, no. 1, 2009, pp. 3-8.

111 Ackerl K, Atzmueller M, Grammer K. "The Scent of Fear." *Neuro Endocrinol Lett.* 2002 Apr;23(2):79-84.

112 https://www.mayoclinic.org/drugs-supplements/tretinoin-topical-route/side-effects/drg-20066521?p=1. Accessed December 23, 2023.

113 https://www.mayoclinic.org/drugs-supplements/benzoyl-peroxide-topical-route/side-effects/drg-20062425?p=1#:~:text=Serious skin reactions (eg, skin,during treatment with this medicine. Accessed December 23, 2023.

114 https://www.mayoclinic.org/drugs-supplements/clindamycin-topical-route/side-effects/drg-20063064

115 https://www.mayoclinic.org/drugs-supplements/spironolactone-oral-route/side-effects/drg-20071534?p=1#:~:text=Check with your doctor right,or heaviness of the legs. Accessed December 23, 2023.

116 Bright E. *Good Fat Is Good For Women: Menopause.*

117 Grigg-Spall H. *Sweetening the Pill: Or How We Got Hooked on Hormonal Birth Control.* John Hunt Publishing, 2013.

118 Bright E. *Good Fat Is Good For Women: Menopause.*

SIX
HOW TO PREVENT AND ADDRESS HEALTH ISSUES DURING PUBERTY AND ADOLESCENCE

1 Doufas AG, Mastorakos G. "The Hypothalamic-Pituitary-Thyroid Axis and the Female Reproductive System." *Ann N Y Acad Sci.* 2000;900:65.

2 Shen J, Cunha GR, Sinclair A, Cao M, Isaacson D, Baskin L. "Macroscopic Whole-Mounts of the Developing Human Fetal Urogenital-Genital Tract: Indifferent Stage to Male and Female Differentiation." *Differentiation.* 2018 Sep-Oct;103:5-13.

3 Nutt, Amy Ellis (14 September 2017). "Wonder Woman Lived: Viking Warrior Skeleton Identified as Female, 128 Years after its Discovery." The Washington Post. ISSN 0190-8286. Archived from the original on 17 September 2017. Retrieved 16 September 2017.

4 Ibid.

5 K. Hawkes. "Grandmothers and Human Evolution." Margo Wilson Memorial Lecture, McMaster University, Hamilton, October 03, 2013

6 Mystery of diseases of ancient Mesopotamians 21.02.2014, https://scienceinpoland.pl/en/news/news,399197,mystery-of-diseases-of-ancient-mesopotamians.html. Accessed November 6, 2023.

7 Roberts, C. (2015). "What Did Agriculture Do for Us? The Bioarchaeology of Health and Diet." In G. Barker & C. Goucher (Eds.), *The Cambridge World History* (The Cambridge World History, pp. 93-123). Cambridge: Cambridge University Press.

8 Snape, Erin. (2012). "Health Impacts at the Advent of Agriculture." *Agricultural and Food Sciences, Environmental Science, History, Medicine.*

9 Haeusler M, Grunstra NDS, Martin RD, Krenn VA, Fornai C, Webb NM. "The Obstetrical Dilemma Hypothesis: There's Life in the Old Dog Yet." *Biol Rev Camb Philos Soc.* 2021 Oct;96(5):2031-2057.

10 Hochberg Z, Gawlik A, Walker RS. "Evolutionary Fitness as a Function of Pubertal Age in 22 Subsistence-Based Traditional Societies." *Int J Pediatr Endocrinol.* 2011;2011(1):2.

11 Wells JC, DeSilva JM, Stock JT. The obstetric dilemma: an ancient game of Russian roulette, or a variable dilemma sensitive to ecology? Am J Phys Anthropol. 2012;149 Suppl 55:40-71.

12 Frost P. "Vitamin D Deficiency Among Northern Native Peoples: A Real or Apparent Problem?" *Int J Circumpolar Health.* 2012 Mar 19;71:1800

13 Merewood A, Mehta SD, Chen TC, Bauchner H, Holick MF. "Association Between Vitamin D Deficiency and Primary Cesarean Section." *J Clin Endocrinol Metab.* 2009 Mar;94(3):940-5.

14 Barker, Graeme; Goucher, Candice (2015). *The Cambridge World History* || What did agriculture do for us? The bioarchaeology of health and diet. , 10.1017/CBO9780511978807(4), 93–123.

15 Ibid.

16 Masclans A, Hamon C, Jeunesse C, Bickle P. "A Sexual Division of Labour at the Start of Agriculture? A Multi-Proxy Comparison Through Grave Good Stone Tool Technological and Use-wear Analysis." *PLoS One.* 2021 Apr 14;16(4):e0249130.

17 Manning Richard. *How Agriculture Hijacked Civilization.* North Point Press, 2004

18 Masclans A, Hamon C, Jeunesse C, Bickle P. "A Sexual Division of Labour at the Start of Agriculture? A Multi-Proxy Comparison Through Grave Good Stone Tool Technological and Use-wear Analysis." *PLoS One.* 2021 Apr 14;16(4):e0249130

19 Diamond, Jared. "The Worst Mistake in Human History." *Discover Magazine*, 1987. http://public.gettysburg.edu/~dperry/Class%20Readings%20Scanned%20Documents/Intro/Diamond.PDF.

20 Love HJ, Sulikowski D. "Of Meat and Men: Sex Differences in Implicit and Explicit Attitudes Toward Meat." *Front Psychol.* 2018 Apr 20;9:559.

21 Işık Balcı Y, Karabulut A, Gürses D, Ethem Çövüt I. "Prevalence and Risk Factors of Anemia among Adolescents in Denizli, Turkey." *Iran J Pediatr.* 2012 Mar;22(1):77-81.

22 Bukachi, S.A., Ngutu, M., Muthiru, A.W. *et al.* "Gender and Sociocultural Factors in Animal Source Foods (ASFs) Access and Consumption in Lower-Income Households in Urban Informal Settings of Nairobi, Kenya." *J Health Popul Nutr* 41, 30 (2022).

23 Bullough V, Voght M. "Women, Menstruation, and Nineteenth-Century Medicine." *Bull Hist Med.* 1973 Jan-Feb;47(1):66-82.

24 Bukachi, S.A., Ngutu, M., Muthiru, A.W. *et al.* "Gender and Sociocultural Factors in Animal Source Foods (ASFs) Access and Consumption in Lower-Income Households in Urban Informal Settings of Nairobi, Kenya." *J Health Popul Nutr* 41, 30 (2022).

25 Avakian A, Haber B. *From Betty Crocker to Feminist Food Studies: Critical Perspectives on Women and Food: Feminist Food Studies: A Brief History.* University of Massachusetts Press, 2005.

26 Ritzel C, Mann S. "The Old Man and the Meat: On Gender Differences in Meat Consumption across Stages of Human Life." *Foods.* 2021 Nov 15;10(11):2809.

27 Frost, P. (2016). "To Supplement or Not to Supplement: Are Inuit Getting Enough Vitamin D?" *Études Inuit Studies* 40(2), 271–291.

28 Narchi H, El Jamil M, Kulaylat N. "Symptomatic Rickets in Adolescence." *Arch Dis Child.* 2001 Jun;84(6):501-3.

29 Gentile C, Chiarelli F. "Rickets in Children: An Update." *Biomedicines.* 2021 Jun 27;9(7):738.

30 Petroski W, Minich DM. „Is There Such a Thing as 'Anti-Nutrients'? A Narrative Review of Perceived Problematic Plant Compounds." *Nutrients.* 2020 Sep 24;12(10):2929.

31 Kårlund A, Paukkonen I, Gómez-Gallego C, Kolehmainen M. "Intestinal Exposure to Food-Derived Protease Inhibitors: Digestion Physiology- and Gut Health-Related Effects." *Healthcare* (Basel). 2021 Aug 5;9(8):1002.

32 Lynch, Lauren. "Treatment of Anemia during Pregnancy (1931), by Lucy Wills". *Embryo Project Encyclopedia* (2017-04-20). ISSN: 1940-5030.

33 Wills L. "Treatment of 'Pernicious Anaemia of Pregnancy' and 'Tropical Anaemia'." *Br Med J.* 1931 Jun 20;1(3676):1059-64.

34 Ibid.

35 Mitchell HK, Snell EE, Williams RJ. Journal of the American Chemical Society, Vol. 63, 1941: The concentration of "folic acid" by Herschel K. Mitchell, Esmond E. Snell, and Roger J. Williams. Nutr Rev. 1988 Sep;46(9):324-5.

36 Leung AM, Braverman LE, Pearce EN. "History of U.S. Iodine Fortification and Supplementation." *Nutrients.* 2012 Nov 13;4(11):1740-6.

37 Kocher ET. "Concerning Pathological Manifestations in Low-Grade Thyroid Diseases." Nobel Lecture, 1909.

38 Leung AM, Braverman LE, Pearce EN. "History of U.S. Iodine Fortification and Supplementation." *Nutrients.* 2012 Nov 13;4(11):1740-6.

39 Marine D. "Prevention and Treatment of Simple Goiter." *Atl. Med. J.*, 26:437-442, 1923.

40 Means J.H., Thomas C.C. "The Function of the Thyroid Gland." American Lecture Series. Publication Number 40., 1949

41 Salter, W.T. *The Endocrine Function of Iodine.* Harvard University Press, 1940, Cambridge, Mass., pg 254-255, 261, 268-269.

42 Biber FZ, Unak P, Yurt F. "Stability of Iodine Content in Iodized Salt." *Isotopes Environ Health Stud.* 2002 Jun;38(2):87-93.,

43 Wang GY, Zhou RH, Wang Z, Shi L, Sun M. "Effects of Storage and Cooking on the Iodine Content in Iodized Salt and Study on Monitoring Iodine Content in Iodized Salt." *Biomed Environ Sci.* 1999 Mar;12(1):1-9.

44 Boothby W.M. "The Use of Iodine in Exophthalmic Goiter." *Clinical Metabolism*, Mayo Clinic. 1924.

45 Abraham, G.E. "The Wolff-Chaikoff Effect: Crying Wolf?" *The Original Internist*, 12(3):112-118, 2005.

46 Calsolaro V, Pasqualetti G, Niccolai F, Caraccio N, Monzani F. "Thyroid Disrupting Chemicals." *Int J Mol Sci.* 2017 Dec 1;18(12):2583.

47 Vishniakova YY, Murav'eva NI. [On the treatment of dyshormonal hyperplasia of mammary glands.] [Article in Russian] *Vestn Akad Med Nauk SSSR* 1966;21(9):19–22.

48 Soldin OP. "Controversies in Urinary Iodine Determinations." *Clin Biochem.* 2002 Nov;35(8):575-9.

49 https://www.hakalalabs.com/The-Many-Types-of-Iodine-Testing_b_4.html. Accessed December 23, 2023.

50 Nolan LA, Windle RJ, Wood SA, Kershaw YM, Lunness HR, Lightman SL, Ingram CD, Levy A. "Chronic Iodine Deprivation Attenuates Stress-Induced and Diurnal Variation in Corticosterone Secretion in Female Wistar Rats." *J Neuroendocrinol.* 2000 Dec;12(12):1149-59.

51 Calsolaro V, Pasqualetti G, Niccolai F, Caraccio N, Monzani F. "Thyroid Disrupting Chemicals." *Int J Mol Sci.* 2017 Dec 1;18(12):2583.

52 "Function in Neonates and Children: A Systematic Review of the Literature." *Nutrients.* 2022; 14(1):168.

53 Abraham, Guy E., Jorge D. Flechas and John Hakala. "Orthoiodosupplementation: Iodine Sufficiency of the Whole Human Body." Environmental Science, Medicine. (2007).

54 Means J.H., Thomas C.C. "The Function of the Thyroid Gland." American Lecture Series. Publication Number 40., 1949

55 Kurilo LF. Follikulogenez v prenatal'nom periode razvitiia cheloveka [Folliculogenesis in the prenatal period of human development]. *Arkh Anat Gistol Embriol.* 1980 Aug;79(8):63-9. Russian.

56 Labrie, "DHEA and the Intracrine Formation of Androgens and Estrogens in Peripheral Target Tissues: Its Role during Aging." *Steroids* vol. 63, n. 5–6, 1998, p. 322-328.

57 Ibid.

58 Enayatjazi M, Sadeghi Dinani S, Emami Hashemi SA. "The Effect of Intensive Exercise on Beta-Endorphin and Serum Cortisol Levels in Elite Wrestlers." *Physical Treatments.* 2015; 5(3):171-176

59 Buske-Kirschbaum A, von Auer K, Krieger S, Weis S, Rauh W, Hellhammer D. "Blunted Cortisol Responses to Psychosocial Stress in Asthmatic Children: A General Feature of Atopic Disease?" *Psychosom Med.* 2003 Sep-Oct;65(5):806-10.

60 Blumberg, Joan Jacobs. *The Fasting Girls.* New York, NY: Plume, 1989.

61 Ibid.

62 Ibid.

63 Prete A, Yan Q, Al-Tarrah K, Akturk HK, Prokop LJ, Alahdab F, Foster MA, Lord JM, Karavitaki N, Wass JA, Murad MH, Arlt W, Bancos I. "The Cortisol Stress Response Induced by Surgery: A Systematic Review and Meta-Analysis." *Clin Endocrinol* (Oxf). 2018 Nov;89(5):554-567.

64 Ball R, Howlett T, Silverstone T, Rees L. "The Interrelationship of Beta Endorphin, ACTH and Cortisol in Depressive Illness: A Controlled Study." *Psychol Med.* 1987 Feb;17(1):31-7.

65 Enayatjazi M, Sadeghi Dinani S, Emami Hashemi SA. "The Effect of Intensive Exercise on Beta-Endorphin and Serum Cortisol Levels in Elite Wrestlers." *Physical Treatments.* 2015; 5(3):171-176.

66 Pilozzi A, Carro C, Huang X. "Roles of β-Endorphin in Stress, Behavior, Neuroinflammation, and Brain Energy Metabolism." *Int J Mol Sci.* 2020 Dec 30;22(1):338.

67 Buske-Kirschbaum A, von Auer K, Krieger S, Weis S, Rauh W, Hellhammer D. "Blunted Cortisol Responses to Psychosocial Stress in Asthmatic Children: A General Feature of Atopic Disease?" *Psychosom Med.* 2003 Sep-Oct;65(5):806-10

68 Metz S, Duesenberg M, Hellmann-Regen J, Wolf OT, Roepke S, Otte C, Wingenfeld K. "Blunted Salivary Cortisol Response to Psychosocial Stress in Women with Posttraumatic Stress Disorder." *J Psychiatr Res.* 2020 Nov;130:112-119.

69 https://www.thecut.com/2020/03/teen-beauty-influencers-are-using-anti-aging-skin-care.html. Accessed December 22, 2023.

70 Sesta A, Cassarino MF, Tapella L, Castelli L, Cavagnini F, Pecori Giraldi F. "Effect of Retinoic Acid on Human Adrenal Corticosteroid Synthesis." *Life Sci.* 2016 Apr 15;151:277-280.

71 S. Jung [et al.] "Dietary Fat Intake During Adolescence and Breast Density Among Young Women." *Cancer Epidemiology, Biomarkers & Prevention* vol. 25, n. 6, 2016, p. OF1-OF10.

72 C. Nagata [et al.] "Association of Dietary Fat, Vegetables and Antioxidant Micronutrients with Skin Ageing in Japanese Women." *British Journal of Nutrition* vol. 103, n. 10, 2010, p.1493-1498.

73 Shoeb A, Chowta M, Pallempati G, Rai A, Singh A. "Evaluation of Antidepressant Activity of Vanillin in Mice." *Indian J Pharmacol.* 2013 Mar-Apr;45(2):141-4.

74 Bradbury J, Meyers S, Oliver. "Are Low-Fat Diets Associated with Stress?" *International Journal of Naturopathic Medicine*, 2004.

75 Venkatraman JT, Feng X, Pendergast D. "Effects of Dietary Fat and Endurance Exercise on Plasma Cortisol, Prostaglandin E2, Interferon-Gamma and Lipid Peroxides in Runners." *J Am Coll Nutr.* 2001 Oct;20(5):529-36

76 Abraham, Guy E., Jorge D. Flechas and John Hakala. "Orthoiodosupplementation: Iodine Sufficiency of the Whole Human Body." Environmental Science, Medicine. (2007).

77 Woodford, Keith. *Devil in the Milk: Illness, Health and the Politics of A1 and A2 Milk*. Chelsea Green Publishing, 2009.

78 Bressan P, Kramer P. "Bread and Other Edible Agents of Mental Disease." *Front Hum Neurosci*. 2016 Mar 29;10:130.

79 Ibid.

80 Ibid.

81 Hockey M, Aslam H, Berk M, Pasco JA, Ruusunen A, Mohebbi M, Macpherson H, Chatterton ML, Marx W, O'Neil A, Rocks T, McGuinness AJ, Young LM, Jacka FN. "The Moo'D Study: Protocol for a Randomised Controlled Trial of A2 Beta-Casein Only Versus Conventional Dairy Products in Women with Low Mood." *Trials*. 2021 Dec 11;22(1):899.

82 Bath SC, Hill S, Infante HG, Elghul S, Nezianya CJ, Rayman MP. "Iodine Concentration of Milk-Alternative Drinks Available in the UK in Comparison with Cows' Milk." *Br J Nutr*. 2017 Oct;118(7):525-532.

83 Caprio AM, Umano GR, Luongo C, Aiello F, Dello Iacono I, Palumbo S, Miraglia Del Giudice E, Grandone A. "Case Report: Goiter and Overt Hypothyroidism in an Iodine-Deficient Toddler on Soy Milk and Hypoallergenic Diet." *Front Endocrinol* (Lausanne). 2022 Aug 11;13:927726.

84 Fomon, S.J. "Iodine and Soy Milk." *Am J Dis Child*. 1962;103(1):97–98.

85 https://www.thetimes.co.uk/article/women-who-eat-little-meat-and-dairy-put-their-health-at-risk-says-scientist-ch2dz0z58.

86 Evershed, R.P., Davey Smith, G., Roffet-Salque, M. et al. "Dairying, Diseases and the Evolution of Lactase Persistence in Europe." *Nature* 608, 336–345 (2022).

87 Schofer, Gill. "G. Stanley Hall: Male Chauvinist Educator." *The Journal of Educational Thought*, vol. 10, no. 3, 1976, pp. 194-200.

88 Graebner W. "'Back-fire to lust': G. Stanley Hall, Sex-Segregated Schooling, and the Engine of Sublimation." *Hist Psychol*. 2006 Aug;9(3):236-246

89 Salk RH, Hyde JS, Abramson LY. "Gender Differences in Depression in Representative National Samples: Meta-Analyses of Diagnoses and Symptoms." *Psychol Bull*. 2017 Aug;143(8):783-822.

90 Figueira, Maria Luisa. "Gender-Related Endocrinological Dysfunction and Mental Disorders." *Current Opinion in Psychiatry* (2010): n. pag. Print.

91 Rubinow, D (2002). "Hormones, Brain and Behavior." Volume Five || *Gonadal Hormones and Behavior in Women Concentrations versus Context.* , (), 37–73.

92 Young EA, Korszun A. "The Hypothalamic-Pituitary-Gonadal Axis in Mood Disorders." *Endocrinol Metab Clin North Am.* 2002 Mar;31(1):63-78.

93 Hooda J, Shah A, Zhang L. "Heme, an Essential Nutrient from Dietary Proteins, Critically Impacts Diverse Physiological and Pathological Processes." *Nutrients.* 2014 Mar 13;6(3):1080-102.

94 Suneson, Klara; Asp, Marie; Träskman-Bendz, Lil; Westrin, Åsa; Ambrus, Livia; Lindqvist, Daniel (2019). "Low Total Cholesterol and Low-Density Lipoprotein Associated with Aggression and Hostility in Recent Suicide Attempters." *Psychiatry Research*, 273(), 430–434.

95 Anita H. Payne, Dale B. Hales. "Overview of Steroidogenic Enzymes in the Pathway from Cholesterol to Active Steroid Hormones." Endocrine Reviews, Volume 25, Issue 6, 1 December 2004, Pages 947–970.

96 Baynham R, Weaver SRC, Rendeiro C, Veldhuijzen van Zanten JJCS. "Fat Intake Impairs the Recovery of Endothelial Function Following Mental Stress in Young Healthy Adults." *Front Nutr.* 2023.

97 Bradbury J, Meyers S, Oliver. "Are Low-Fat Diets Associated with Stress?" *International Journal of Naturopathic Medicine*, 2004.

98 Venkatraman JT, Feng X, Pendergast D. "Effects of Dietary Fat and Endurance Exercise on Plasma Cortisol, Prostaglandin E2, Interferon-Gamma and Lipid Peroxides in Runners." *J Am Coll Nutr.* 2001 Oct;20(5):529-36

99 Grosso G, Galvano F, Marventano S, Malaguarnera M, Bucolo C, Drago F, Caraci F. "Omega-3 Fatty Acids and Depression: Scientific Evidence and Biological Mechanisms." *Oxid Med Cell Longev.* 2014;2014:313570.

ABOUT THE AUTHOR

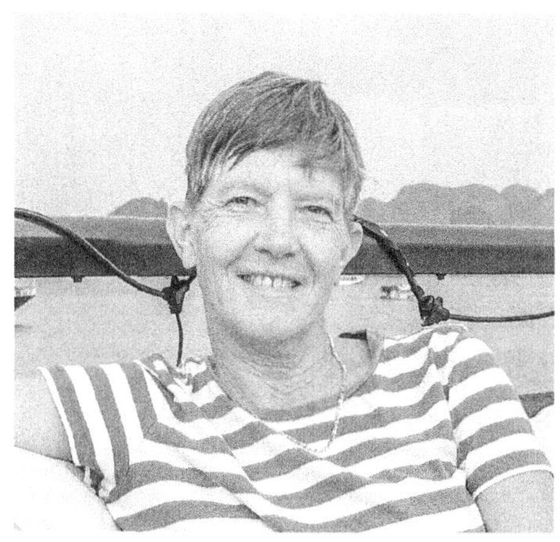

Elizabeth Bright DO, ND, (New York 1963) is an American osteopath and naturopath using diet to optimize endocrine function. She is a former chef, a master in traditional Cha Ka Kung Fu, an avid stand-up paddleboarder, and fluent in several languages. She divides her time between Italy and Scotland. Dr. Elizabeth Bright is the author of *Good Fats Is Good for Women: Menopause.*

www.ElizBright.com

Printed in Great Britain
by Amazon